Adult Development
and Well-Being:
The Impact
of Institutional Environments

Adult Development and Well-Being: The Impact of Institutional Environments has been co-published simultaneously as *Journal of Human Behavior in the Social Environment,* Volume 15, Number 4 2007.

Adult Development and Well-Being: The Impact of Institutional Environments

Catherine N. Dulmus, PhD
Karen M. Sowers, PhD
Editors

Adult Development and Well-Being: The Impact of Institutional Environments has been co-published simultaneously as *Journal of Human Behavior in the Social Environment*, Volume 15, Number 4 2007.

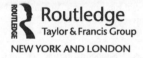

Routledge
Taylor & Francis Group

NEW YORK AND LONDON

Adult Development and Well-Being: The Impact of Institutional Environments has been co-published simultaneously as *Journal of Human Behavior in the Social Environment,* Volume 15, Number 4 2007.

The development, preparation, and publication of this work has been undertaken with great care. However, the publisher, employees, editors, and agents of The Haworth Press and all imprints of The Haworth Press, Inc., including The Haworth Medical Press® and Pharmaceutical Products Press®, are not responsible for any errors contained herein or for consequences that may ensue from use of materials or information contained in this work. Opinions expressed by the author(s) are not necessarily those of The Haworth Press, Inc. With regard to case studies, identities and circumstances of individuals discussed herein have been changed to protect confidentiality. Any resemblance to actual persons, living or dead, is entirely coincidental.

The Haworth Press is committed to the dissemination of ideas and information according to the highest standards of intellectual freedom and the free exchange of ideas. Statements made and opinions expressed in this publication do not necessarily reflect the views of the Publisher, Directors, management, or staff of The Haworth Press, Inc., or an endorsement by them.

First published by
The Haworth Press, Inc., 10 Alice Street, Binghamton, NY 13904-1580

This edition published 2014 by Routledge
711 Third Avenue, New York, NY 10017, USA
2 Park Square, Milton Park, Abingdon, Oxon OX14 4RN

Routledge is an imprint of the Taylor & Francis Group, an informa business

Library of Congress Catalog-in-Publication Data

Adult development and well-being: the impact of institutional environments / Catherine N. Dulmus, Karen M. Sowers, editors.
  p. cm.
  "The Impact of Institutional Environments has been co-published simultaneously as Journal of Human Behavior in the Social Environment, Volume 15, Number 4 2007."
  Includes bibliographical references and index.
  ISBN 978-0-7890-3646-9 (hard cover : alk. paper) – ISBN 978- 0-7890-3647-6 (soft cover : alk. paper)
  1. Adulthood–Social aspects. 2. Social institutions. 3. Social service. I. Dulmus, Catherine N. II. Sowers, Karen M. (Karen Marlaine) III. Journal of human behavior in the social environment.

  HQ799.95.A36 2008
  305.240973–dc22   2007045720

Adult Development and Well-Being: The Impact of Institutional Environments

CONTENTS

ABOUT THE EDITORS

Catherine N. Dulmus, PhD, is Associate Professor and Director of the Buffalo Center for Social Research in the School of Social Work at the University at Buffalo. She received her baccalaureate degree in Social Work from Buffalo State College in 1989, the master's degree in Social Work from the University at Buffalo in 1991 and a doctoral degree in Social Welfare from the University at Buffalo in 1999. As a researcher with interests in school and community violence and children's mental health, Dr. Dulmus' recent contributions have focused on fostering interdependent collaborations among practitioners, researchers, schools, and agencies critical in the advancement and dissemination of new and meaningful knowledge. She has authored or coauthored several journal articles and books, and has presented her research nationally and internationally. Dr. Dulmus is co-editor of *The Journal of Evidence-Based Social Work: Advances in Practice, Programming, Research, and Policy*, co-editor of *Best Practices in Mental Health: An International Journal*, associate editor of *Stress, Trauma, and Crisis: An International Journal*, and sits on the editorial boards of the *Journal of Human Behavior in the Social Environment, Victims and Offenders, Journal of Evidence-Based Policies and Practices,* and *Journal of Health and Social Policy*. Prior to obtaining the PhD her social work practice background encompassed almost a decade of experience in the fields of mental health and school social work.

Karen M. Sowers, PhD, was appointed Professor and Dean of the College of Social Work at the University of Tennessee, Knoxville in August 1997. She served as Director of the School of Social Work at Florida International University from June 1994 to August 1997 and as the Undergraduate Program Director of the School of Social Work at Florida International University from 1986 to 1994. She received her baccalaureate degree in Sociology from the University of Central Florida in 1974, the Master's Degree in Social Work from Florida State

University in 1977 and the PhD in Social Work from Florida State University in 1986. Dr. Sowers serves on several local, national and international boards including the Council on Social Work Education Commission on Curricular Innovation and Excellence, the International Planning Committee for the International Consortium for Social Development, the American Board of Mental Health Examiners, and the International Task Force on Social Work Education of the National Association of Deans of Social Work. Dr. Sowers is nationally known for her research and scholarship in the areas of international practice, juvenile justice, child welfare, cultural diversity and culturally effective intervention strategies for social work practice, evidence-based social work practice and social work education. Her current research and community interests include evidence-based practice, mental health practice, international social work practice and juvenile justice practice. She has authored or co-authored numerous books, book chapters and refereed journal articles. She has served as a founding editorial board member of the *Journal of Research on Social Work Practice*, founding co-editor of *Best Practices in Mental Health: An International Journal* and is currently serving on the editorial boards of the *Journal of Evidence-Based Social Work: Advances in Practice, Programs, Research and Policy* and *Journal of Stress, Trauma and Crisis: An International Journal.*

Preface

Institutions serving adults can positively or negatively impact adult development and subsequently outcomes on well-being. This may include those outcomes which would facilitate reintegration into community and society as well as individual well-being within an institutional setting. This volume is devoted to examining that impact and how we can improve outcomes for adults whose adult development is impacted by institutional policy and service delivery. This collection conceptualizes "institutions" across methods (individual, family, group, community and organizations) and across populations and problems providing a broad perspective on the impact of institutions on the functioning of adults across the life span. The eight articles demonstrate the outstanding work in our field to move practice forward in improving outcomes for clients. Given the Council on Social Work Education's (CSWE) strengthened emphasis in this area, the editors hope that the compilation of this research provides meaningful data for social work education programs and subsequent social work practice with adults in institutional settings.

The lead article by Bunch, Eastman and Moore, is timely as it addresses military deployment and its impact on grandparents who step into a full time child care role with grandchildren as a result of parental deployment. Their descriptive study examines the experiences of 23 grandmothers who report problematic levels of stress as well as changes in both intimate and social relationships as a result of their new child caring roles. The second article by Curtiss, Hayslip and Dolan reports a study of 75 institutionalized older adults as to the impact of length of residence, gender, voluntariness and motivational style on indicators of adjustment to long-term institutionalization. The third article by Farone and Pickens reports on qualitative data from interviews with twenty people who identified as having serious mental illness to identify how the mental health system impacts their sense of self.

[Haworth co-indexing entry note]: "Preface" Co-published simultaneously in *Journal of Human Behavior in the Social Environment* (The Haworth Press, Inc.) Vol. 15, No. 4, 2007, pp. xxi-xxii; and: *Adult Development and Well-Being: The Impact of Institutional Environments* (ed: Catherine N. Dulmus, and Karen M. Sowers) The Haworth Press, Inc., 2007, pp. xvii-xviii. Single or multiple copies of this article are available for a fee from The Haworth Document Delivery Service [1-800-HAWORTH 9:00 a.m. - 5:00 p.m. (EST). E-mail address: docdelivery@haworthpress.com].

Available online at http://jhbse.haworthpress.com
© 2007 by The Haworth Press, Inc. All rights reserved.
doi:10.1300/J137v15n04

The fourth article by Critelli focuses on low-income foster mothers and the additional challenges welfare reform policies have created for them. The study explores care-giving as an important aspect of gender and cultural identity and survival strategy for these foster mothers and provides policy recommendations to reduce the negative aspects that this social institution has on low-income foster mothers. The next article by Rowe reminds us that in many situations, for individuals that are institutionalized, normal sexual development is disrupted by among other things lack of privacy, gender separated living environment, lack of sex education, and lack of opportunity. Recognizing that all people whatever their circumstances are sexual beings, Rowe advocates for the need of explicit institutional policies that provide an atmosphere where sexual expression can be normalized as much as possible while ensuring a safe and supportive environment. The sixth article by Bunch, Eastman and Griffin examines the life satisfaction perceptions of grandparents who parent in formal and informal kinship care arrangements due to the child's biological parents being no longer able to provide a stable environment. Also included is an article by McCarter who looks at the impact of hopelessness and hope on social service workers related to burnout and the organizational characteristics that contribute to it.

The final article is a very thoughtful essay authored by Miller who argues that the U.S. Census is an institution that influences U.S. law and public policy, subsequently impacting adult development through the distribution of privilege between Whites and Nonwhites.

The research highlighted in this collection represents important contributions on the impact of institutions on adult development and well-being. Across the various social institutions discussed in this special issue potentially negative and positive impacts on adult development could be attributed to institutional settings or systems. It is the editors' hope that this volume will spur further interest and research in this area. The development and dissemination of knowledge specific to the impact of institutions on outcomes for adults is of paramount importance. Institutions affect large numbers of adults and their families. It is critical to the well-being of communities and society, as well as the individual, that we recognize that institutions do indeed impact adult development and thus work to develop practice and policy strategies that reduce negativity and increase pro-social functioning over the lifespan.

Catherine N. Dulmus, PhD
Karen M. Sowers, PhD
Editors

A Profile of Grandparents Raising Grandchildren as a Result of Parental Military Deployment

Shelia Grant Bunch
Brenda J. Eastman
Robin Rene Moore

SUMMARY. There is a growing number of grandparents faced with the need to raise their grandchildren as a result of the military deployment of their own child. This is a descriptive study that examines the experiences of 23 grandmothers who are providing full time child care

Shelia Grant Bunch earned her PhD from North Carolina State University. She is a member of the faculty at East Carolina University's School of Social Work. Dr. Bunch has extensive experience in working children and families in health care settings and victims of family violence in rural localities. Her research interests include family violence, child welfare, kinship care and maternal and child health and social work practice in rural settings.

Brenda J. Eastman obtained her PhD from Virginia Commonwealth University's School of Social Work. She is now a member of the faculty at The School of Social Work in East Carolina University. Dr. Eastman has provided clinical services to adolescent sex offenders and their families for over 15 years and continues to be interested in clinical work with offender populations. Her research interests include youthful offenders, family violence, child welfare, and child development.

Robin Rene Moore is a graduate student at East Carolina University.

Address correspondence to: Shelia Grant Bunch, School of Social Work, Room 116 Ragsdale Hall, Greenville, NC 27858 (E-mail: bunchs@ecu.edu).

[Haworth co-indexing entry note]: "A Profile of Grandparents Raising Grandchildren as a Result of Parental Military Deployment." Bunch, Shelia Grant, Brenda J. Eastman, and Robin Rene Moore. Co-published simultaneously in *Journal of Human Behavior in the Social Environment* (The Haworth Press, Inc.) Vol. 15, No. 4, 2007, pp. 1-12; and: *Adult Development and Well-Being: The Impact of Institutional Environments* (ed: Catherine N. Dulmus, and Karen M. Sowers) The Haworth Press, 2007, pp. 1-12. Single or multiple copies of this article are available for a fee from The Haworth Document Delivery Service [1-800-HAWORTH, 9:00 a.m. - 5:00 p.m. (EST). E-mail address: docdelivery@haworthpress.com].

Available online at http://jhbse.haworthpress.com
doi:10.1300/J137v15n04_01

to their grandchildren. Results suggest that these grandparents are experiencing problematic levels of stress as well as changes in both intimate and social relationships. doi:10.1300/J137v15n04_01 *[Article copies available for a fee from The Haworth Document Delivery Service: 1-800-HAWORTH. E-mail address: <docdelivery@haworthpress.com> Website: <http://www. HaworthPress.com> © 2007 by The Haworth Press, Inc. All rights reserved.]*

KEYWORDS. Grandmothers, grandchildren, military, stress

INTRODUCTION

The separation of military members from their families has been an increasingly common experience for military families. Statistics from the Department of Defense (2006) indicate that at the present time, approximately 350,000 women are serving in the U.S. military representing almost 15 percent of active duty personnel. In the past the role of women in the military has been limited in scope to non-combat positions which precluded them from specific types of jobs. The repeal of Title 10 U.S. Code, section 6015 authorized the Secretary of Defense to change military personnel policy to assign women to any combat unit, classes of combat vessels, and combat platforms (SECNAV Instruction 1300.12c, N13W, 28 Dec 2005). Since the repeal of the "combat exclusion law" a greater number of women are serving than ever before with women representing one in every seven military personnel assigned in Iraq. In addition, 35 women soldiers have died as of March 2005, and 261 U.S. military women have been wounded in Iraq.

Although researchers have explored the impact of deployment of the male military member on families, the research on the impact the deployment of military women have on the family is limited at best (Kelly, Hock, Jarvis, Smith, Gaffney, & Bonney, 2002). In an ethnography of U.S. Navy women's experiences of deployment, Navy mothers reported greater levels of anxiety and guilt over having their career obligations compromise their role as parents (Kelly, Herzog-Simmer, & Harris, 1994). Wynd and Dziedzicki (1992) reported that women during operation Desert Storm experienced greater levels of separation anxiety and guilt over being unable to parent their children then their male counterparts. Military parents may experience difficulty managing their roles as worker and parent and may require much assistance for balancing their military careers with family life.

A number of studies have looked at the impact of parental deployment on military children. One of the first studies that examined the impact of father absence on children described increases in anxiety and depression among children of deployed military personnel as compared to non-deployed military personnel (Jensen, Lewis, & Xenakis, 1989). After interviewing children of military personnel deployed in Desert Storm, Peebles-Kleiger, and Kleiger (1994) reported that children in families experiencing parental deployment at times of war are at a higher risk of experiencing symptoms of post traumatic stress disorder than children of parents in a non-war deployment assignment. As of January 2005, over 1400 service members have been killed in Operation Iraqi Freedom, resulting in over 900 children losing their parents and to date, there have been no studies conducted related to the parenting of these children (Cozza, Chun, & Polo, 2005).

As a result of work-related separation, military parents are often unable to serve as primary caregivers to their children. As a result, grandparents may be asked to provide care and assistance to their grandchildren (Kelly et al., 2002). The phenomenon of grandparents being placed in the capacity of primary caregivers has been one that has gained much attention in the literature over the past decade. According to U.S. Census data, 2.4 million children were living with grandparent caregivers and 39% of grandparent caregivers had cared for their grandchildren for 5 or more years (U.S. Census Bureau, 2003). The psychological consequences of this event are numerous. In instances where military parents seek parental care from their own parents, the grandparent is often placed in a situation where care giving has to take place in the shadow of losing their own child. As a result they are likely to question whether or not they are competent enough to deal with raising children again (Pinson-Millburn, Fabian, Schlossberg, & Pyle, 2001).

Grandparents may feel overwhelmed with negotiating their own physical and emotional needs in addition to the needs of their grandchildren. Grandparents who assume custodial care of grandchildren have to manage and coordinate the legal, medical, educational and social service needs of their grandchildren. (Kelly, Yorker, Whitley, & Sipes, 2001). The lifestyles and daily routines of grandparents are interrupted and dreams and aspirations for retirement are often deferred (Dowdell, 1995; Sands & Goldberg-Glen, 1998). Grandparents may not be able to meet the physical demands of parenting due to pre-existing health problems or their health deteriorates after assuming care (Landry, 1999; Musil, 1998) because they do not interrupt their care giving responsibilities to seek health care for themselves.

The psychological well-being of grandparents may also impact their ability to adequately coordinate care for their grandchildren (Szinovacz,

DeViney, & Atkinson, 1999; Minkler & Roe, 1993). Kelly, Whitley, Sipe, and Yorker (2000) found that 30% of their sample reported psychological distress scores in the clinical range resulting from limited resources, lack of support and poor physical health. Mental health issues faced by grandparents in general tend to stem from the lifestyle negotiations they make to incorporate full time care giving into their daily routine. Psychological stress and anxiety are exacerbated by the inability of many grandparents to sustain relationships with social and community networks and they often report a loss of freedom and social isolation (Minkler, Fuller-Thomson, Miller, & Driver, 1997; Musil, 1998).

The tasks of grandparenting when parents are deployed are myriad. The grandparents have to cope with the duality of managing their own anxiety about the safety and well-being of their children as well as helping their grandchildren cope with the anxiety about the safety of their parents (Cozza et al.) In addition, the grandparents must help the grandchildren cope with the disruption of their normal routines exacerbated by relocation to reside with their grandparents, adjusting to new schools and establishing a new social network of friends. Grandparents will have to establish a parental role with their children to include the establishment of disciplinary rules and boundaries. Grandparents may need to establish a sense of normalcy for their grandchildren that may be counterintuitive to their own daily routines (Arana-Barradas, 2004).

Even though the deployed parent may have completed a Family Care Plan in preparation for deployment, the transition can be stressful for all involved. A comprehensive Family Care Plan includes provisions for financial, legal, medical and social care of minor children during parental deployment and separation. The grandparents may experience less stress when the deployed military member has completed a comprehensive plan. The lack of a comprehensive plan or an incomplete plan will instigate numerous problems and concerns for grandparents by increasing their probability of negotiating legal, educational and social service systems that may be unfamiliar to them (http://magellanassist.com). Grandparents often have to negotiate aging and, child welfare, school, health care and legal systems which are different and often confusing social service systems. Each of these systems have their own bureaucratic rules, policies and funding (Roe, 2000). Legal issues may emerge when grandparents have physical custody of their grandchildren but do not have legal custody, thereby, increasing the frustration of enrolling children school, daycare and sports activities or obtaining medical and dental care (Heywood, 2001).

While there have been studies of the impact of military deployment on military dependent mothers and children, there have not been any studies the impact on custodial grandparents. The purpose of this research is to explore the impact of military deployment on grandparents in light of the growing number of women with children in the military. These grandparents may not qualify for public assistance or other social service programs, therefore, the needs of this small unique population of grandparents may be obscured. These grandparents are dually impacted by military deployment because they have to endure the anxiety of coping with the safety and well-being of two generations of family members.

METHOD

Participants

A non-probability purposive sampling technique was utilized to recruit participants for the survey. Investigators identified organizations hosting support groups for grandparents raising their grandchildren in localities near military installations in North Carolina and Virginia and then contacted the administrative personnel in each organization. Once contacted, the purpose of the study, target population, study procedures were explained and agency cooperation in recruiting potential participants was solicited. Written information was then forwarded to cooperating agencies so that potential participants could be told about the study. An investigator would then visit the agency, meet with the potential participant and again provide information about the goals of the study, the role of the survey interview, and request participation. Upon the indication of consent, a direct contact protocol was implemented. The recruitment of participants took place over a six month interval and yielded a sample size of 23 grandparents whose adult children were on military deployment and as a result were now in the position of being the primary caregiver for their grandchildren.

Measures

The instrument used in this study was a multi-faceted questionnaire, comprised of a brief questionnaire developed by the investigators and three self report instruments, assessing participant satisfaction with life, personal stress, satisfaction with parenting. The study questionnaire gathered demographic information about the care giver and their perceptions about whether providing care has had an impact on their health or inter-personal relationships. Table 1 provides a summary of interview questions and participant responses.

The Satisfaction with Life Scale (Diener, Emmons, Larsen, & Griffin, 1994) is comprised of five items assessing the cognitive-judgmental aspects of general life satisfaction. Unlike measures that apply some external standard, the Satisfaction with Life Scale (SWLS) reveals the individual's own judgment of his or her quality of life. Respondents read each statement and respond using a 7 point Likert Scale ranging from "strongly disagree" to "strongly agree." Item scores are summed for a total score, which ranges from 5 to 35, with higher scores reflecting more satisfaction with life. The authors report that the SWLS's internal consistency is very good, with an alpha of .87 and a good test-retest reliability with a correlation of .82 for a two month period. Concurrent validity was tested with samples varying adult samples reflecting young and older adult populations, while the authors reported that scores correlated with nine measures of subjective well-being, not further data was provided.

The Index of Clinical Stress (Abell,1994) is a 25-item instrument designed to measure the degree or magnitude of problems clients have with personal stress. The items were designed to reflect the range of perceptions associated with subjective stress. Respondents respond to each statement using a 7-point Likert Scale. A score is calculated that can range from 0 to 100 with the higher scores indicating greater magnitude or severity of problems. The Index of Clinical Stress (ICS) has excellent internal consistency, with an alpha of .96. The author reports the ICS as having good factorial validity and construct validity.

The Kansas Parental Satisfaction Scale (Schumm & Hall, 1994) is a 3 item instrument designed to measure satisfaction with oneself as a parent, the behavior of one's children, and a person's relationship with the child. Items are rated using a 7 point Likert scale, responses are summed and can range from 3 to 21 with higher scores indicating satisfaction with one's parenting. The Kansas Parental Satisfaction Scale (KPS) has very good internal consistency, with alphas that range from .78 to .85.

RESULTS

Descriptive Findings

The grandparents who were interviewed became caregivers of their grandchildren as a consequence of their child's military deployment and ranged in age from 54 to 66, with a mean of 60.5 years. Over 65% of

TABLE 1. Demographic Characteristics and Questionnaire Responses (N = 23)

Item	n	%
Race		
Caucasian	8	34.7
African American	15	65.3
Marital Status		
Married	14	61.4
Divorced	6	26.1
Never married	2	8.6
Widowed	1	4.3
Employment		
Working full-time	13	56.4
Retired	7	30.4
Social Security	3	13.0
Do you think your health status has changed		
Yes	19	82.5
No	4	17.5
Self report on health status		
Very Good	0	0
Good	8	34.8
Fair	11	47.7
Poor	4	17.5
Has care giving impacted your relationship with partner		
Yes	14	60.8
No	0	0.0
Not Applicable	9	39.1
Has care giving had an impact on your social network		
Yes	21	91.4
No	2	8.6
Custody Status		
Has Legal Custody	8	34.8
Has Guardianship or temporary custody	11	47.7
No change made prior to deployment	4	17.5
Number of Children being cared for		
One	19	82.7
Two	3	13.0
Three	1	4.3

the grandmothers were African American while the remaining study participants were Caucasian. Sixty-one percent (61%) of the grandparents were married, 26% were divorced, 9% reported that they were never married, and the remaining 4% were widowed. The majority (82%) of the grandparents were providing care for one grandchild. The a little over half of the participants reported that their income was derived from full time employment (56%). All participants reported receiving a monthly allotment from their adult military child in order to assist with child rearing.

Of the participants who were married, all of them reported a change in their relationship with their partner since taking on the responsibility of caring for their grandchildren. Reasons for these changes included: having less privacy than before care giving, having less time to spend with their partner, experiencing more disagreements about child rearing practices, and changes in both the way leisure time is spent together as well as the amount of leisure time together. In addition to viewing changes in their intimate relationships, over 90% of all of the study participants reported that caring for their grandchildren had impacted their social network. The most frequent change experienced by the participants was the reduction of time spent with friends engaged in leisure or recreational activities. Participants reported feeling like they had less time to go out socially with other persons in their age category. They also relayed that they had less time to be involved in social activities associated with church or community groups which they had been involved in prior to assuming care. While participants reported that they felt their friends supported their new role as primary care provider, their new role made them feel more distant or isolated from their circle of friends.

The issue of custody status of the grandchildren appeared to fall into three categories. Thirty-five percent (35%) of the participants reported having legal custody of their grandchildren. The remaining members of the sample reported having some type of temporary arrangement made such as guardianship or a temporary custody agreement or had no arrangements made. Those participants with either temporary custody or guardianship stated that they had experienced some difficulty in resolving issues requiring proof of custody, such as arranging daycare, school enrollment, or health care. The participants who had not negotiated any changes in custody relayed that they had not really given much thought to the possible issues they would have to address. Many of these participants expressed their hope that the deployed parent would return to assume custody soon and that they would not be in a situation where the question of custody became an issue.

The majority of participants reported that they had experienced a change in their health status since taking on the care of their grandchildren. Only 35% of the grandmothers reported their perception of their health status as good, almost half (48%) viewed their health status as fair, and the remaining members of the study saw their health status as poor. No one reported their health status as being very good.

In looking at the three self report instruments, group scores did not indicate severe problems or issues with stress or perceived satisfaction with life. Scores for the Satisfaction with Life Scale ranged from 12 to 31 with a mean score of 24.5 and a standard deviation of 2.22. The Scale's authors reported a norm of 25.8 for an elderly population. While the study's participant group scores were lower, the difference was not significant $t(21) = 1.23, p = .198$. Scores on the Index of Clinical Stress ranged from 48 to 82, with a mean of 60.8 and a standard deviation of 15.6. While Abell (1994), did not report a specific norm for an elderly population, a mean score of 28.9 (SD = 18.7) was reported for an instrument norm. When comparing the author's reported scale mean with the group mean of the study participants, the difference in scores was observed to be significant $t(21) = 9.21, p < .000$. The reported participant mean score of 60.8 indicates that members of this study were experiencing problems with stress. Participant scores for the Kansas Parental Satisfaction Scale ranged from 8 to 15, with a mean of 13.2 (SD = 3.7). The Scale's author reports a norm score of 17.4 (SD = 2.20) for a parental sample in their forties. In a comparison of group means, a significant difference was again observed ($t[21] = 6.45, p < .000$), the grandparents in the study reported lower levels of satisfaction with themselves as parents as compared to parents in populations studied when the author constructed the instrument.

The relationship between the self report instruments and variables from the study questionnaire was examined. Table 2 contains a correlation matrix comprised of variables observed to have a significant relationship. The SWLS was observed to have a strong inverse correlation with both the ICS and KPS. Other variables showing significant relationships with the self report instruments include health status, social network, custody, and marital status.

DISCUSSION

This was a descriptive study of 23 grandparents who were caring for their grandchildren as a result the of military deployment of their parents. One of the greatest stressors that military families experience is separation due to deployment. Those stressors are compounded in

TABLE 2. Intercorrelations for Satisfaction with Life Scale (SWLS) Index of Clinical Stress (ICS), Kansas Parental Satisfaction Scale (KPS) and Selected Survey Responses

Measure	1	2	3	4	5	6	7
1. SWLS	–						
2. ICS	–.49	–					
3. KPS	.68	–.43	–				
4. Health Status	.83	.54	.87	–			
5. Social Network	.45	–.73	–.44	.78	–		
6. Custody Status	.55	.66	.42	.33	.52	–	
7. Marital Status	.72	.65	.59	.33	.44	.52	–

All values observed to be significant $p < .01$

instances where the parent being deployed is the primary child care provider and alternative child care arrangements are made with extended family members (Pittman, Kerpelman, & MacFadyen, 2004). As of this date, there is a paucity of research on how deployment impacts grandparents who assume care of their grandchildren. This study sought to address this deficit through examining the experiences of a small group of grandparents whose adult children are deployed, leaving them in the position of parenting once again. These grandparents share many similarities with other grandparent groups caring for grandchildren, reporting changes in their relationships with partners, social networks (Sands, Goldberg-Glen, & Thornton, 2005). What appears to separate this group from much of the literature on kinship care is the absence of a direct link to the institution responsible for making them parents again. In cases of formal kinship care, the care giver has direct contact with personnel within the child welfare system. While the military offers many services for its members and their immediate families, there are no provisions for services to grandparents caring for military dependents (Cozza, Chun, & Polo, 2005).

The findings of this study need to be interpreted cautiously and several limitations should be noted. The sample is small and reflects a very specialized population, parents of military service personnel with young children. Participant responses to the study's questionnaire are subject to personal biases and distortions characteristic of self-administered surveys. The survey instrument was constructed by the authors for the study; therefore issues of reliability and validity remain. Thus, conclusive statements about grandparents caring for grandchildren when their parents are deployed cannot be made. Information in this study indicates that a grandparent's satisfaction with life is directed impacted by marital status, custody status of the child involvement in social networks and health status. Of particular concern are findings suggesting that this population experiences significant levels of clinical stress. However, more research is needed to better delineate what mediating variables play the largest role in caregiver perceptions and experiences.

This study undoubtedly raises more questions than it answers. How are children affected by living with grandparents when their parents are deployed? How are grandparents affected when they resume parenting responsibilities as a result of the deployment? How do grandparents cope with the changes in their lifestyle that accompanies their new responsibilities? How do the stressors of grandparents affect the well-being of the grandchildren? What support systems if any are in place to assist grandparents? Future research endeavors should further investigate these questions in light of increased deployment trends of military members.

REFERENCES

Abell, N. (1994). Index of Clinical Stress. In J. Fischer & K. Corcoran (Eds.) *Measures for Clinical Practice, Volume 2* (pp. 281-282). New York, NY: The Free Press.

Arana-Barradas, L.A. (2004) The children left behind. *Airmen, 48*(11), 36-41.

Cozza, S.J., Chun, R.S., & Polo, J.A. (2005). Military Families and Children during Operation Iraqi Freedom. *Psychiatric Quarterly, 76*, 371-378.

Deiner, E., Emmons, R., Larson, R.J., & Griffin, S. (1994). Satisfaction with Life Scale. In J. Fischer & K. Corcoran (Eds.) *Measures for Clinical Practice, Volume 2* (pp. 501-502). New York, NY: The Free Press

Dowdell, E.B. (1995). Caregiver Burden: Grandparents raising their high risk grandchildren. *Journal of Psychosocial Nursing, 33*(3), 27-30.

Heywood, E. (2001). Grandparents raising grandchildren: An exploration of their parenting stress and perceived social support. Dissertation, University of Virgina.

Jensen, P.S., Lewis, R.L., & Xenakis, S.N. (1989). The military family in review: Context, risk, and prevention. *Journal of the American Academy of Child Psychology, 60*, 225-234.

Kelly, M.L., Herzog-Simmer, P.A., & Harris, M.A. (1994). Effects of military induced separation on the parenting stress and family functioning of deployed mothers. *Military Psychology, 6*, 125-138.

Kelly, M.L., Hock, E., Jarvis, M.S., Smith, K., Gaffney, M.A., & Bonney, J.F. (2002). Psychological adjustment of Navy mothers experiencing deployment. *Military Psychology, 14*(2), 199-216.

Kelly, S.J., Yorker, B.C., Whitley, D.M., & Sipe, T.A. (2001). A multimodal intervention for grandparents raising grandchildren: Results of an exploratory study. *Child Welfare, 80*(1), 27-50.

Kelly, S.J., Whitley, D., Sipe, T.A., & Yorker, B.C. (2000). Psychological distress in grandmother kinship care providers: The role of resources, social support and physical health. *Child Abuse & Neglect, 24*(3), 311-321.

Landry, L. (1999). Research into action: Recommended intervention strategies for grandparent caregivers. *Family Relations, 48*(4), 381-390.

Military family readiness: The family care plan. http://www.magellanassist.com/mem/librarydefault.asp?topicID=2002&CategoryID=0&ArticleId=55. Retrieved on March 13, 2006.

Minkler, M., & Roe, K. (1993). Grandmothers as caregivers: Raising the children of the crack cocaine crisis. Newbury Park, CA: Sage Publications.

Minkler, M., Fuller-Thomson, E., Miller, D., & Driver, D. (1997). Depression in grandparents raising grandchildren. *Archives of Family Medicine, 6*, 445-452.

Musil, C. (1998). Health, stress, coping and social support in grandmother caregivers. *Health Care for Women International, 19*(5), p. 441, 15 pages.

Pearlin, L. I., & Schooler, C. (1978). The structure of coping. *Journal of Health and Social Behavior, 19*(1), 2-21.

Pinson-Millburn, N., Fabian, E., Schlossberg, N., & Pyle, M. (1996). Grandparents raising grandchildren. *Journal of Counseling and Development, 74*, 548-554.

Pittman, J.F., Kerpelman, J.I., & MacFadyen, J.M. (2004). Internal and external adaptation in army families: Lessons from Operation Desert Shield and Desert Storm. *Family Relations, 53*, 249-260.

Roe, K. (2000). Community interventions to support grandparent caregivers: Lessons learned from the field. In Carole Cox (Ed.) *To grandmother's house we go and stay: Perspectives on custodial grandparents.* Springer Publishing Co: New York: NY.

Sands, R.G., & Goldberg-Glen, R.S. (1998). The impact of employment and serious illness on grandmothers who are raising their grandchildren. *Journal of Women & Aging, 10*(3), 41-58.

Schumm, W.R., & Hall, J. (1994). Kansas Parental Satisfaction Scale. In J. Fischer & K. Corcoran (Eds.) *Measures for Clinical Practice, Volume 1* (pp. 345-346). New York, NY: The Free Press.

Szinovacz, M.E., DeViney, S., & Atkinson, M.P. (1999). Effects of surrogate parenting on grandparents' well-being. *Journals of Gerontology, 54B*(6), S376-S388.

U.S. Census Bureau (2003). Grandparents living with grandchildren: 2000. www.census.gov/prod/2003pubs/ck-31.pdf. Retrieved 11-14-05.

Whitley, D.M., Kelley, S.J. & Sipe, T.A. (2001). Grandmothers raising grandchildren: Are they at increased risk of health problems? *Health and Social Work, 26*(2), 105-114.

Wynd C.A., & Dziedzicki, R.E. (1992). Heightened anxiety in Army reserve nurses anticipating mobilization during Operation Desert Storm. *Military Medicine, 157*, 630-634.

doi:10.1300/J137v15n04_01

Motivational Style, Length of Residence, Voluntariness, and Gender as Influences on Adjustment to Long Term Care: A Pilot Study

Karin Curtiss
Bert Hayslip, Jr.
Diana C. Dolan

SUMMARY. Seventy-five institutionalized older adults (M age = 79.08, SD = 9.73, 25 males, 50 females) varying by length of residence, gender, and motivational style (self determined vs. motivational) were queried to explore the impact of these variables on indicators of adjustment, i.e., health, life satisfaction, desired and expected control, self-esteem, ADLs, and positive/negative affect. MANCOVAs (controlling for social desirability) indicated self-determined motivational style to positively impact adjustment, as well as to interact ($p < .05$) with gender in this respect. Length of residence and gender each impacted ADLs, and motivational style also affected both desired/expected control and self-esteem, where those with higher self determined motivational styles had expectations for

Karin Curtiss, PhD, Bert Hayslip, Jr., PhD, and Diana C. Dolan, BS, are all affiliated with the Department of Psychology, University of North Texas, Denton, TX.

Address all correspondence to Bert Hayslip, Jr., PhD, at the Department of Psychology, P.O. Box 311280, University of North Texas, Denton, TX 76203-1280.

[Haworth co-indexing entry note]: "Motivational Style, Length of Residence, Voluntariness, and Gender as Influences on Adjustment to Long Term Care: A Pilot Study." Curtiss, Karin, Bert Hayslip, Jr., and Diana C. Dolan. Co-published simultaneously in *Journal of Human Behavior in the Social Environment* (The Haworth Press, Inc.) Vol. 15, No. 4, 2007, pp. 13-34; and: *Adult Development and Well-Being: The Impact of Institutional Environments* (ed: Catherine N. Dulmus, and Karen M. Sowers) The Haworth Press, 2007, pp. 13-34. Single or multiple copies of this article are available for a fee from The Haworth Document Delivery Service [1-800-HAWORTH, 9:00 a.m. - 5:00 p.m. (EST). E-mail address: docdelivery@haworthpress.com].

doi:10.1300/J137v15n04_02

and desirability of control. Voluntariness of the decision to move generally positively impacted adjustment, but its impact was moderated by motivational style. Thus, persons who vary along motivational style, gender, voluntariness, and length of residence are likely to function in distinct ways in adjusting to being institutionalized. doi:10.1300/J137v15n04_02

[Article copies available for a fee from The Haworth Document Delivery Service: 1-800-HAWORTH. E-mail address: <docdelivery@haworthpress.com> Website: <http://www. HaworthPress.com> © 2007 by The Haworth Press, Inc. All rights reserved.]

KEYWORDS. Older adults, institutionalization, motivation, gender, adjustment

INTRODUCTION

Relocation from a previous residence to a nursing home is without doubt a period of adjustment for many older persons and their families. In this light, numerous variables may impact such adjustment in that different people adjust differently to placement in a nursing home for different reasons. While there exists much research on adjustment as it relates to older adults with dementia (e.g., Meehan, Robertson, & Vermeer, 2001) or to older persons with mental illness (e.g., Brandt, Campodonico, Rich, Baker, Steele, Ruff, Baker, & Lyketsos, 1998), and while older persons may adjust differently to nursing home relocation in relation to these variables, all older persons face some common challenges with regard to relocation.

Adjustment to a nursing home requires coping with the demands of an environment in which one has never before resided. New residents must learn to adapt to this environment and may be affected by the quality of their relationship with staff, which may be undermined by attrition (Hogstel, 2001). Indeed, during the transition into the nursing home, certain changes may become apparent to either the staff, the resident, or the resident's family. For example, during the first few months of residence in a nursing home, both a decline in overall cognitive status as well as a decline in affective expression as observed by others has been documented (Krichbaum, Ryden, Snyder, Pearson, Hanscom, Lee, & Savik, 1999). It is important to note that not all work supports the association of cognitive change and adjustment to institutional living per se (O'Connor & Vallerand, 1998), wherein relocation to a nursing home environment may simply unmask such changes that were either ignored or not previously recognized by family or friends. In addition, nursing home residents may become more vulnerable to the stress of "deteriorating health, loss of family friends [and] familiar activities" than other older adults in the context of this new environment (O'Connor & Vallerand). To this extent, older individuals relocating to a nursing home may therefore experience a higher level of stress than those who do not relocate, wherein the degree of perceived difference between one's prior residence and this new environment in the nursing home influences subjective levels of stress (Mikhail, 1992). Because older adults who hold control expectations of an internal nature react more positively when they have more control (Moos, 1981), they may adjust more poorly to the structured environment of the nursing home than older adults whose expectation of control is external in nature. Moreover, the relocation effect of the move into a nursing home, where those who have poor psychological adjustment have a heightened probability of death within four years, has been observed (O'Connor & Valleran). In this context then, adjusting to relocation in a nursing home can clearly have potentially disastrous consequences for older persons.

Because not all older persons respond to relocation in the same manner, knowledge of those factors differentiating older persons in this context is key to the planful transition from one's home to a long-term care facility. One factor that may affect adjustment to the nursing home environment is motivational style. O'Connor and Vallerand (1994) found that motivational style, or the motivation to engage in everyday behavior within the context of the freedom to do so, was associated with varying degrees of successful adjustment among a sample of older adults residing in a nursing home, where individuals with a self-determined motivational style adjusted better when their nursing home environment allowed for more freedom of choice (O'Connor & Vallerand). However, this style was not beneficial for individuals whose motivational style was non-self-determined; such individuals adjust better to an environment that provides for fewer choices (O'Connor & Vallerand).

Intuitively, one might expect that adjustment would improve with increased exposure to an environment. A perusal of the literature, however, reveals that there is very little work that has included length of residence in relation to nursing home adjustment. A study by Bowsher and Gerlach (1990) found that length of stay was predictive of adjustment (1990), and more recently, it was found that from admission to six months post-admission, satisfaction with the nursing home remained the same or increased, but did not decrease (Krichbaum, Ryden, Snyder, Pearson, Hanscom, Lee, & Savik, 1999).

For some older adults, the decision to relocate to a nursing home may not be a voluntary one. Some families cannot physically care for an older relative, or may not be able to provide the care necessary to deal with certain health problems, leaving the older person little choice but to move into a residential facility. In this context, the importance of perceived choice in the decision to relocate to a group home was underscored in a study of rural aged persons, who felt that the voluntariness of their decision significantly affected their adjustment to the new environment (Armer, 1996), wherein voluntary relocation was a positive factor in adjustment. Indeed, perceived control over the decision to relocate was found to have positive effects on health during the first month of residency (Davidson & O'Connor, 1990). Importantly, however, perceived voluntary relocation also had negative effects on both health and morale from the second to the fourth months of residency, and thus, voluntariness of relocation may negatively impact adjustment in the long term (Davidson & O'Connor). This work suggests that no consensus exists regarding the impact of voluntariness of relocation on nursing home adjustment.

Gender differences also appear to impact adjustment to a nursing home. In one study which examined the relationship between length of residence and adjustment in light of possible gender differences (Claridge, Rowell, Duffy, & Duffy, 1995), results showed that while length of stay was a positive predictor of nursing home satisfaction among males, no such relationship existed for females (Claridge et al.). A more recent study found that gender was one of three characteristics which accounted for the variance in ratings of satisfaction with the nursing home environment (Krichbaum, Ryden, Snyder, Pearson, Hanscom, Lee, & Savik, 1999), where men were generally less likely to experience adjustment problems than were women, and tended to report less dissatisfaction with the nursing home (Greenwood, 1999). Thus, there are likely gender differences that may interact with other variables, i.e., voluntariness and length of residence in affecting nursing home adjustment.

Our goal in this paper is to explore the joint effects of motivational style, length of residence, and voluntariness of the decision to relocate as these factors relate to nursing home adjustment, and to investigate any possible gender differences in such relationships. As older adults entering the nursing home environment frequently experience lessened control over many aspects of their daily lives, of particular interest in this regard are such effects on perceptions of both desired and expected control, as well as self-esteem, activities of daily living (ADLs), and positive affect.

At the minimum, it was expected that persons with a style that was generally more non-self-determined would have better adjustment than those with a more self-determined style (at least in the nursing home environment), and that length of stay would generally positively influence adjustment, and that adjustment would be generally superior for women than for men.

METHOD

Participants

Seventy-five institutionalized older adults with a mean age of 79.08 ($SD = 9.73$) defined the sample in the present study. A third of the sample was male ($n = 25$) and two thirds were female ($n = 50$), paralleling the make-up of the older population (see Hayslip & Panek, 2002) as well as the census in most long-term care facilities (see Hogstel, 2001). Seventy-two were Caucasian. Over half of participants had at least a high school education (56%), while the other 44% had up to 24 years of formal education ($M = 12.81$, $SD = 3.74$). The majority of participants were widowed (74.7%), 12% were still married, 9.3% were either divorced or separated, and only 4% had never been married. Sixty-four percent had living children, and 70% had living grandchildren. Almost half (41.3%) had lived in a nursing home prior to their current place of residence. For a large number of residents, the decision to relocate to a nursing home was either completely voluntarily or made with some consultation (65.3%), whereas 34.7% perceived themselves to have had little or no control over relocation. The remaining residents (21.4%) reported that they were consulted in the relocation decision, but did not make the decision themselves. Residents had lived in the nursing home for an average of 14.55 months [SD = 18.72, Range = 0 (newly admitted) to 96 months].

Procedure

Potential volunteers were identified in consultation with the nursing staff, wherein the first and second authors had first been granted access to the facility by the nursing home administrator. Informed consent forms that were signed by both the older adult and a witness were typed in a large font and were read to participants as needed. Volunteers who did not attain a score of higher than 15 on the short form of the Mini-Mental

State exam (see below) (Folstein, Anothy, Parhad, Duffy, & Gruenberg, 1985) or were unable to physically participate were subsequently excluded from the study. In addition, volunteers had to be older than 65 to participate. Participants were then interviewed by either the primary investigator or a graduate student assistant, wherein participants completed under supervision standardized measures assessing a variety of constructs relevant to the present study (see below). If necessary, such items were read to the resident and he or she responded verbally to each.

Measures

Mini-Mental State Exam

The Mini Mental State Exam(MMSE) is a brief measure of cognitive function (Folstein, Folstein, & McHugh, 1975), and was used to screen potential volunteers prior to their involvement in the study (see above). The abbreviated version used here consisted of nine items that measure orientation to time and place, attention, memory, and language skills. A maximum of 24 points are possible, with higher scores indicating higher levels of cognitive functioning. Among a sample of depressed and demented elderly adults with stable clinical histories, test-retest reliability after 28 days was .98 (Folstein et al.). Correlations of .78 for the Verbal IQ and .66 for the Performance IQ of the Wechsler Adult Intelligence Scale (WAIS) establish the MMSE's concurrent validity (Folstein et al.). Generally speaking, evidence for the MMSE's sensitivity and specificity is extensive (Langley, 2000).

Elderly Motivation Scale

The Elderly Motivation Scale (EMS) is a 13-item measure of motivational style (Vallerand & O'Connor, 1991). In this study, participants were asked to respond to each question by rank ordering (where 1 = most important and 4 = least important) four choices representing a different motivational style, ranging from amotivational (I don't know, I don't see what it does for me), non-self-determined extrinsically motivated (Because I am supposed to do it), self-determined extrinsically motivated (For the pleasure of doing it), to intrinsically motivated (I choose to do it for my own good). Internal consistency reliability ranges from .88 to .89 (Vallerand & O'Connor) for each. When items were categorized as either self-determined or non-self-determined, as might be expected, the correlation between the two motivational styles was highly negative ($r = -.824, p < .01$). In this light, for this study, the four choices were combined to define a single continuum, ranging from a self-determined/internal style, encompassed by items defining self-determined (both extrinsically and intrinsically) motivated persons, to a non-self-determined/external style, encompassed by items defining amotivational and non-self-determined (extrinsically) motivated persons. Items dealt with topics such as one's activities in light of health, physical self-care, seeing one's doctor, maintaining relationships with family and friends, practicing one's religion, engaging in recreational activity, and following the news. For purposes of defining levels of motivational style in this study, persons were dichotomized as falling above or below the sample median, and responses were recoded for each style such that persons falling below the median (greater rated importance) for the self-determined style and above the median (lesser rated importance) for the non-sclf-dctermined style were classified as "internal." In contrast, persons falling below the median (greater rated importance) for the non-self-determined style and above the median (lesser rated importance) for the non-self-determined style items were classified as "external."

Activities of Daily Living

The Activities of Daily Living Questionnaire (ADL) consists of six items asking participants to rate the level of assistance required to complete that activity (Katz, Ford, Moskowitz, Jackson, & Jaffe, 1963). Higher scores on this measure indicate the need for more assistance with ADLs. Overall correlations with Raven's matrices and a range of motion test indicate evidence of its concurrent validity (Katz, Downs, Cash, & Grotz, 1970 as cited in Ernst & Ernst, 1984). The Katz et al. index of ADLs is noted as the measure of ADL performance upon which all other measures have been built (Pearson, 2000); both self-ratings and staff ratings were collected in this study.

Marlowe-Crowne Social Desirability Scale

The brief version of the Marlowe-Crowne Social Desirability Scale (M-C 1) was utilized here, and consists of ten items (Strahan & Gerbasi, 1972). Half of the items when answered with a true response and half of the items when answered with a negative response indicate when the participant attempts to respond in a socially favorable manner. Correlations with the full version of the scale range from the .80s to .90s (Strahan & Gerbasi).

Affect Balance Scale

The Affect Balance Scale (ABS) consists of two subsets of five questions measuring positive and negative affect during the past few weeks (Bradburn, 1969). Persons respond yes or no to each item. The total score is computed by subtracting the sum of the negative subset from the sum of the positive subset, and higher such scores indicate greater general psychological well-being. Test-retest reliability after three days is .76 for the combined scale, .81 for the negative affect subscale (NAS), and .83 for the positive affect subscale (PAS; Bradburn). The ABS has been found to correlate positively ($r = .61$) with a measure of morale among older persons (Moriwaki, 1974).

Self Esteem Scale

The Self-Esteem Scale (SES) is a ten item measure assessing participants' feelings of self-worth (Rosenberg, 1965). Subjects respond using a four-point Likert-type scale, with possible total scores ranging from 10 to 40. The SES has an internal consistency reliability of .88 (Fleming & Courtney, 1984) and a test-retest reliability of .85 over a two-week interval (Silber & Tippett, 1965, as cited in Blascovich & Tomaka, 1991). There is a correlation of .65 between the SES and self-rated confidence but only a correlation of .39 between SES and popularity (no p-value given; Lorr & Wunderlich, 1986).

Life Satisfaction Index Z

The Life Satisfaction Index Z (LSI-Z) is a 13 item measure of general contentment and happiness (Wood, Wylie, & Sheafor, 1969). For each item, persons endorse either agreement, disagreement, or "don't know." Wood, Wylie, and Sheafor found the Kuder-Richardson reliability for the LSI-Z to be .79. The LSI-Z is positively correlated ($r = .57, p < .01$) with the Life Satisfaction Ratings scale, which measures contentment and positive self-regard (Lohmann, 1977).

Desired Control Measure

The Desired Control Measure (DCM) consists of two subsets of 35 items relating to desired and expected control on a five point Likert-type scale ranging from Very Undesirable to Very Desirable and Strongly Disagree to Strongly Agree, respectively (Reid & Ziegler, 1981). In this study, a short form (two 16-item subsets) was utilized. Internal consistency for the short form ranges from .69 to .74 (Reid & Zeigler). The DCM-Short Form is positively correlated ($r = .42$, $p < .001$) with the Subjective Senescence measure (Reid & Zeigler), and has been shown to be sensitive to the effects of retirement preparation training and related to retirement attitudes (Abel & Hayslip, 1986, 1987).

Participants were also asked to rate their current health compared to others of their own age as very poor, poor, fair, or good. Higher scores indexed poorer self-perceived health. They were also asked to rate the extent to which they thought the move was voluntary, where higher such scores indicated *less* perceived voluntariness (ranging from 1 = entirely voluntary/under one's control to 4 = completely involuntary/beyond one's control).

RESULTS

Data Analysis

Factor Structure of Dependent Variables

In light of the relative smallness of the sample, which generally speaking, detracted from the statistical power of the analyses, and given the attenuated degrees of freedom associated with an analysis of each of the above separate scales singly or as a set, the above measures (except for social desirability response bias) were subjected to a principal components analysis with varimax rotation to a terminal solution, whose purpose was to derive a composite index of adjustment that would be more reliable than that associated with each of the above measures. This analysis, where the subjects to variables ratio was 9:1, yielded a three-factor solution, wherein the principal components so derived were orthogonal to one another (see Tabachnick & Fidell, 1996), and which collectively accounted for 67.6% of the common variance among the above measures of adjustment. Based upon the rotated principal component (PC) matrix solution so derived, PC scores were saved and utilized in the analyses reported below.

The three principal components derived were principally defined (using a criterion of .40 or above, loadings for each in parentheses) by (1) lower scores on negative affect (–.747), and higher ADL (–.602), self esteem (.826), life satisfaction (.583), and greater expectancy of control scores (.770), accounting for 39.1% of the common variance among measures (Eignevalue = 3.13), and labeled here as General Adjustment (PC1), (2) higher scores on positive affect (.888) and life satisfaction (.596), secondarily defined by better health (−.337), and labeled here as Positive Emotion (PC2), accounting for 15.5% percent of the measures' common variance (Eigenvalue = 1.24) and (3) poorer ratings of health (.635) and greater desirability of control (.771), secondarily defined by more negative affect (.294), and labeled here as Passive Control (PC3). PC3 accounted for 12.9% of the common variance among the dependent variables (Eigenvalue = 1.04).

Analyses of the Effects of Motivational Style, Length of Residence, and Gender

Utilizing the above principal component scores as dependent variables, a 2 (gender) × 2 (length of residence) × 2 (motivational style–internal versus external) multivariate analysis of covariance (MANCOVA), controlling for social desirability response bias, was performed to explore our expectations regarding the impact of these independent variables on adjustment to institutional residence. As noted above, residents' motivational styles were categorized as either self-determined/internal or non-self-determined/external. Categories of length of stay were defined given its distribution in this sample, wherein approximately one half of the sample had lived in the nursing home for one year or less, so this point was used to divide the sample into two roughly equal groups. The dependent variables in this analysis were the above derived principal component scores (PC1, PC2, PC3), wherein more positive (or less negative) scores reflect better adjustment, and more negative (or less positive) scores indicate less adequate functioning (factor scores are scaled to a mean of 0 and an SD of 1).

Because there were fewer men than women in this sample, the triple interaction between motivational style, gender, and length of stay, as well as the gender by length interaction, could not be tested (only one male had been institutionalized for longer than a year), and thus only main effects and the remaining two-way interactions could be tested here. Findings reported here derived from MANCOVAs reflect adjusted means, taking into consideration the impact of social desirability response bias.

Findings for Principal Component Factor Scores

When levels of self determined/internal motivational style were each explored in concert with length of stay and gender, only main effects for motivational style were statistically significant at the multivariate level, $F_{3,63} = 2.87$, $p < .05$. At the univariate level, main effects for motivational style moderately impacted PC1 (General Adjustment) scores, $F_{1,65} = 3.71$, $p = .058$, favoring those with a self-determined/external style ($M = .042$, $SE = .27$) over those with a non-self-determined style ($M = -.243$, $SE = .17$), contrary to prediction. The impact of motivational style was substantial for PC3 (Passive Control) scores, $F_{1,65} = 4.13$, $p < .05$, but favored those with a non-self-determined style ($M = -.177$, $SE = .17$) over those whose style was self-determined ($M = -.214$, $SE = .28$), consistent with our expectations. The motivational style by gender interaction approached statistical significance for PC3 scores, $F_{1,65} = 3.24$, $p < .08$, wherein among those with a self-determined/external style, PC3 scores for men tended to be lower ($M = -.614$, $SE = .52$) than those for women ($M = .186$, $SE = .19$). Among those with non-self-determined styles, these differences were similarly ordered, but their absolute magnitude was greater (for males, $M = -.627$, $SE = .30$; for females, $M = .054$, $SE = .22$). The main effect for gender was statistically significant for PC3 scores, $F_{1,65} = 4.47$, $p < .04$, with such scores favoring women ($M = .120$, $SE = .15$) over men ($M = -.622$, $SE = .37$).

Findings for Individual Measures of Adjustment

As an exploratory endeavor, when this analysis was replicated utilizing the above measures of adjustment as a set, only length of residence's effects were statistically significant at the multivariate level, $F_{8,58} = 2.09$, $p = .05$; this was unique to ADLs, $F_{1,65} = 6.23$, $p < .02$, where such scores were higher (indicating greater needs for assistance) for those who had resided longer (a year or less, $M = 15.86$, $SE = .56$; more than a year, $M = 19.46$, $SE = 1.39$). At the univariate level, the effect of motivational style was specific to self esteem, $F_{1,65} = 5.60$, $p < .02$, desirability of control, $F_{1,65} = 5.21$, $p < .03$, and expectancy of control, $F_{1,65} = 5.64$, $p < .02$. Self-esteem scores were higher for those with internal motivational styles ($M = 31.29$, $SE = 1.15$ versus $M = 29.33$, $SE = .73$); this was similarly true for both desirability ($M = 69.76$, $SE = 1.60$ versus $M = 68.22$, $SE = 1.01$) and expectancy ($M = 56.39$, $SE = 2.04$ versus $M = 53.41$, $SE = 1.29$) of control scores. Gender differences in ADLs favored women ($M = 16.11$, $SE = .56$) over men ($M = 19.16$, $SE = 1.41$), $F_{1,65} = 4.56$, $p < .04$. The gender by motivational style interaction approached statistical significance for desirability of control, $F_{1,65} = 3.62$, $p < .06$, and indicated that among self-determined older persons, desirability scores were somewhat lower for men ($M = 68.50$, $SE = 3.02$) than for women

($M = 71.03$, $SE = 1.13$). Among non-self-determined persons, men's desirability scores were much lower ($M = 64.91$, $SE = 1.72$) than those for women ($M = 69.88$, $SE = 1.27$).

The Impact of Perceived Voluntariness of the Move

For the entire sample, while length of residence could not be crossed with gender (see above), a voluntariness (where lower scores indexed more perceived voluntariness) by motivational style by gender MANCOVA indicated no effects at the multivariate level for the principal component scores. However, the perceived voluntary nature of the move was moderately (?) associated with better Overall Adjustment (PC1), $F_{1,66} = 3.53$, $p < .06$, ($M = .189$, $SE = .14$ versus $M = -.289$, $SE = .19$), as was a more self-determined motivational style (see above). The voluntariness by motivational style effect was also substantial for PC2, $F_{1,66} = 4.06$, $p < .05$, wherein among those whose style was self-determined and who saw the move as voluntary, PC2 scores were higher ($M = .244$, $SE = .20$ versus $M = -.329$, $SE = .22$), while for those whose style was non-self-determined, findings were reversed, favoring those for whom the move was seen as nonvoluntary ($M = .192$, $SE = .31$ versus $M = -.293$, $SE = .22$).

When this analysis was replicated for the individual measures of adjustment, as above, no multivariate effects emerged. At the univariate level, expectancy of control was moderately impacted by voluntariness, $F_{1,70} = 3.69$, $p = .058$, favoring those for whom the move was seen as voluntary ($M = 56.60$, $SE = 1.07$) over those for whom the move was seen as beyond their control ($M = 53.05$, $SE = 1.51$). In addition, persons who saw the move as voluntary and whose motivational style was self-determined had greater expectations of control, $F_{1,70} = 7.03$, $p < .01$, ($M = 59.23$, $SE = 1.44$ versus $M = 54.20$, $SE = 2.10$). For those who motivational style was non-self-determined, these differences were similarly ordered, but of less magnitude ($M = 53.96$, $SE = 1.58$ versus $M = 51.89$, $SE = 2.18$).

When voluntariness was crossed with motivational style and length of residence, the above effects of voluntariness on PC1 were similar, while the voluntariness by control effect was weakened. However, the voluntariness by length of residence effect was substantial for PC3 (Passive Control), $F_{1,64}$, 4.41, $p < .05$, where such scores were higher ($M = -.003$, $SE = .18$ versus $M = -.157$, $SE = .25$) among persons who viewed the move as voluntary and who had lived in the nursing home for less time. Such effects however, were reversed among persons who viewed the move as beyond their control (residence of a year or less, $M = -.286$, $SE = .25$, versus a more than a year, $M = .654$, $SE = .34$).

For individual measures, the effect of voluntariness on self esteem was statistically significant ($F_{1,65} = 4.42$, $p < .05$), favoring those ($M = 30.84$, $SE = .63$ versus $M = 28.61$, $SE = .86$) who viewed the move as voluntary. Length of residence negatively impacted life satisfaction, $F_{1,65} = 3.86$, $p < .05$, favoring those who had resided for less time ($M = 8.81$, $SE = .51$ versus $M = 7.11$, $SE = .69$). Among those who viewed the move as voluntary and who had resided longer, ADL scores were higher (indicating greater needs for assistance) ($M = 14.88$, $SE = .68$ versus $M = 17.40$, $SE = .96$), $F_{1,65} = 4.20$, $p < .05$. In contrast, for those who saw the move as beyond their control, this pattern was reversed ($M = 17.60$, $SE = .97$ versus $M = 16.04$, $SE = 1.29$). The triple interaction was substantial for Negative Affect, $F_{1,64} = 4.12$, $p < .05$, and indicated that for persons who had self-motivational styles, who saw the move as beyond their control, and who had resided for a longer time, such scores were highest ($M = 3.75$, $SE = .71$). Scores were nearly as high for persons whose style was non-self-determined, who viewed the move as nonvoluntary, and who had resided for less time ($M = 3.34$, $SE = .61$) (all other cell means failed to exceed 2.3).

Individual Differences Analyses

Individual differences in relationship between length of residence, motivational style, and nursing home adjustment were explored via Pearson correlations, computed separately for males and females. Because of the high negative correlation between self-determined and non-self-determined styles ($r = -.824$), only correlations with the self-determined/internal style are reported here. For men, lower self-determined style scores were related to higher PC1 scores ($r = -.560$, $p < .01$); this was true as well for PC3 scores ($r = -.388$, $p < .03$). For women as well, lower self-determined styles were linked to higher PC1 scores ($r = -.289$, $p < .03$), and among women, greater length of residence was weakly related to higher such scores ($r = .189$, $p < .09$). When motivational styles were intercorrelated with specific measures of adjustment for men, greater internality was significantly ($p < .05$) associated with more negative affect ($r = .415$), less self esteem ($r = -.534$), and less desirability of control ($r = -.549$) and to a certain extent, less expectancy of control ($r = -.368$, $p < .07$). For females, greater internality was linked ($p < .05$) to less self-esteem ($r = -.326$) and less expectancy of control ($r = -.286$).

When perceptions of the voluntariness (where higher scored index *less* voluntariness) of the decision was correlated with both principal component scores and individual measures scores for men, no such relationships emerged. For women, more perceived voluntariness was linked ($p < .05$) more self-esteem ($r = -.410$), and more expectancy of control ($r = -.379$), as well as to higher PC1 scores ($r = -.371$).

DISCUSSION

This study investigated nursing home residents' responses to various items chosen to assess several aspects of nursing home adjustment, which is itself a complex, multifaceted construct. Of principal interest here was the impact of motivational style, which is likely to be salient in that many aspects of residents' lives, by virtue of the limitations of their health, or via constraints imposed upon them by institutional policy and routine, especially given the understaffed nature of many facilities and the often unstable pattern of professional and paraprofessional employment over time.

Perhaps most apparent in these findings is the impact of motivational style on adjustment, wherein, generally speaking, those whose styles were more self-determined fared better. Perhaps such a style enabled them to better cope with, and indeed, overcome the routinous nature of institutional life, suggesting they are resilient in this respect. This finding is indeed consistent with the pattern of coping among women labeled active mastery by Guttman (1975). Importantly however, this finding is in contrast with the picture painted by Baltes (1996), who stresses the role of one's having developed a relationship with staff where residents' well-being was contingent upon behaving in a manner that would make them easier to care for. In this context, Baltes and Carstensen (1999) have discussed the "learned dependency," characteristic of many older institutionalized residents, that is a response to the micro-environment of the nursing home culture, fostering dependence to the ignorance of autonomy (see Baltes, 1996). Such persons are said to have developed "excess disabilities" which strengthened their dependence upon staff (Kahn & Miller, 1978). The question becomes one of interpretation; is dependence upon others desirable? These data suggest that if one values his or her own capacity to make independent decisions, then the answer to this question must be "no."

It is important to observe that for some older persons, such styles may reflect the reality that is imposed upon many by being institutionalized, forcing them to come to terms with their own physical limitations. Such persons may have even shifted their style, having been previously more self-determined, though longitudinal data would be necessary to support such a hypothesis. In this light, it is important to observe that Passive Control (PC3) scores indeed favored those with non-self-determined styles. Not surprisingly, the above findings regarding the effect of motivational style, as well as for the motivational style by gender effect were echoed at the level of specific measures of adjustment. Importantly, and in light of the above learned dependence model proposed by Baltes (1996), the style by gender interaction obtained here suggests that such effects have more disadvantageous consequences for men than for women; among men whose styles were more self-determined, PC3 scores were lower, despite the passive nature of PC3 scores. This is also consistent with the fact that desirability of control scores were especially low for men whose motivational styles were non-self-determined, perhaps reflecting the realities of the perceived loss of control in the nursing home, and possibly resulting in futile attempts, i.e., learned helplessness (Seligman, 1975), and/or the appearance of excess disabilities, to control their everyday lives. Among non-self-determined males, their styles might have likely been present for some time prior to entering the nursing home. Alternatively, some may have altered their styles in response to nursing home life. This picture regarding motivational style and its effects varying by gender are generally reinforced via the pattern of intercorrelations reported above separately for men and women. Key here would be longitudinal data speaking to changes in motivational styles over time.

Generally speaking, this inclination to think in certain characteristic ways about the reasons one behaves in the way one does in terms of motivational style seems therefore to be related to multiple indices of nursing home adjustment. Thus, these data suggest that older men whose choices and/or behaviors may be heavily influenced by external sources (i.e., other people or their environment) will not likely make an easier transition into a more restrictive, structured environment such as a nursing home, to the extent that such constraints clash with one's motivational style.

In this respect, it is instructive to discuss the implications of the findings for voluntariness. Indeed, a more subjective, but no less revealing picture of older persons' perceptions of the consequences of being institutionalized is reflected in their views about the voluntariness of the decision to relocate to a nursing home environment. As might be expected, persons who saw the move as under their control fared better regarding their adjustment to institutional life. Interestingly, and in part, in contrast to the findings for motivational style, for those whose perceptions of the move and motivational style were in concert with one another, adjustment outcomes were better. That is, when persons' perceptions of the control over the decision to move are reinforced by the motivational style they have apparently been able to either (a) maintain in the face of institutional life or (b) have developed in response to everyday routines, their adjustment is better, and both their expectation of, and the desirability of having personal control are apparently advantageous to them.

It is of note that ADLs declined with length of residence, as might be expected as persons' health and functional skills worsen over time, consistent with the negative impact of length of residence on life satisfaction. Moreover, the gender difference favoring women for PC3 scores is understandable given the availability of other women as providers of social support, and given the fact that women outlive men, generally speaking (see Hayslip & Panek, 2002; Hogstel, 2001). This finding may also suggest that older women are more successful in adapting to institutional life than are older men. The individual differences findings for women bear this out, especially when such persons see the move as a decision into which they have substantial input.

In a nursing facility, many aspects of daily life (e.g., getting up, meals, baths, activities) are highly regimented and tightly scheduled. If a person can be conceptualized as someone who makes choices in accordance with others' agendas, it is indeed possible that persons whose style is self-determined are more adept at picking up upon the necessity for "fitting in," and therefore fare better in the context of daily living in a nursing home environment. This resident will likely adapt better in making a smoother transition upon moving into a nursing home than someone who tends to make choices less aligned with their own priorities and wishes; this finding has been reported in past work (e.g., O'Connor & Vallerand, 1994).

An interesting question to be raised here is how many persons with a given motivational style have always been inclined to make decisions in this fashion, as opposed to those who have altered their motivational styles upon entering the nursing home, as noted above. That is, what proportion of older persons are naturally motivated by internal resources, and whose attributions for their own behavior are more internalized, versus those who have come to rely more on their environment since entering the facility? In this respect, declines in life satisfaction and ADLs may be at work, as persons naturally become more dependent upon others as their functional skills deteriorate, with apparently negative consequences attached to such changes. In addition, among this second subset of residents, how many have evolved independently and how many have been molded by their surroundings? Given the structure and regimen of many nursing facilities, it is not beyond imagination to suppose that in some cases the nursing home setting "pulls for" a more non-self-determined motivational style, whereas in others that foster more independence, self-determined motivational styles prove advantageous.

A significant interaction was found between voluntariness of the move (the decision to relocate having been made by the resident or another person) and length of residency (one year or less vs. more than one year) in relation to Passive Control and ADLs. When persons made their own decision to move into the nursing facility and length of residency was shorter, Passive Control scores increased, suggesting that they had learned to adapt in a nonassertive manner to nursing home life. Interestingly, and reflecting the realities of institutional life, Passive Control scores were higher among persons who saw the move as involuntary and who had resided for a longer period of time. In this respect, they had indeed overcome their feelings about relocating and were most likely demonstrating learned dependency that was adaptive (Baltes, 1996). Thus, when someone else (e.g., family member of physician) makes the decision to move, residents with a stay of more than one year must learn to cope with their own feelings of helplessness and subsequently use such skills to their advantage over time. Indeed, the triple interaction for Negative Affect highlights the disadvantageous consequences for persons who value control in terms of motivational style and the decision to move. In fact, the Negative Affect data suggest that some persons, despite their externalized orientation to control, nevertheless still have initial adjustment difficulties.

Implications for Nursing Facilities

Increased awareness of the adjustment process and dramatic change in lifestyle associated with relocation to the nursing home is of key importance for the nursing home staff, the family of the new resident, and the resident herself. Advanced preparation by all involved parties could greatly ease the transition that must be made by the resident and her family, especially for men and for persons who view the world from the outside in, wherein greater degrees of support might be necessary. For others, i.e., women, such support may be less crucial, as they may be more adaptive, and may be more successful in imposing themselves on the nursing home environment. Clearly, as the time for the person's move to a nursing home facility draws closer, efforts should be made by individuals responsible for making the decision to learn as much as possible about life at the facility before the relocation actually takes place. While making the decision to relocate, issues such as scheduled wake-up times, meals, baths, and prospective roommates may appear relatively insignificant; this may especially be the case when a concerned family is making arrangements regarding medical services and finances. Helping a prospective resident learn more abut life at the nursing home in advance, however, can make the adjustment easier, simply by making less of her new lifestyle an "unknown." Also, by researching ahead of time, special arrangements may be possible that will make life more tolerable (or even pleasurable) once the move takes place. Examples include leaning about offered activities that the resident enjoys (e.g., such as cards, trivia games, crafts); requesting, specifically if the resident is cognitively alert, that the prospective roommates be at a similar level of functioning; and planning in advance how the resident would like her room to be decorated, along with choosing specific, favorite belongings that she feels comfortable taking with her.

Once the move has occurred, efforts should be made to provide the self-determined resident with as many opportunities as possible to maintain or acquire some control over everyday life, as our data suggest this to be an important facet of overall adjustment. Importantly however, an awareness of the importance of setting visiting times that can be kept consistently, or having choices regarding preferred meals and leisure activities for some residents and not others, is key. In many nursing facilities, residents have an accessible, consistent mechanism through which concerns, grievances, recommendations, and comments may be expressed to the staff; such avenues may or may not be valued by men versus women, or by residents who vary in motivational style.

Clearly, it is critical that staff and family members understand the magnitude of the transition the resident is being required to undergo. In some cases, the person is recovering from a serious illness or injury, which in itself calls for adjustments and/or compromises of some sort. In most instances, the person's functioning has deteriorated to the point that she can longer care for herself independently. Very often, the resident is leaving her own home, which she may have lived in for a large portion of her life, to move into one room which she may be required to share with a complete stranger (who may or may not be someone with whom she can communicate). Finally, it is crucial that the resident's room be respected and treated as that person's home, particularly by staff who come in and out several times daily. When one's home is restricted to such a small area, privacy is of the utmost importance.

Limitations of the Present Study

The major limitations of this study are those associated with the size and characteristics of the sample. Of these 75 interviewees, only twenty-five were men, and of course, the entire sample is self-selected and unique to this particular facility. In addition, almost the entire sample is Anglo-American, so ethnicity was an important demographic characteristic that remained completely unaddressed here. Finally, it is important to note that only the highest functioning residents were interviewed, as due to length and complexity of the interview itself, less highly functioning residents were screened. Thus, generalizations to less functional residents must be made with caution. Other limitations of the study relate specifically to aspects of the interview itself. First, to keep the interview as brief and "respondent-friendly" as possible, some measures were modified. For example, items were eliminated from the Folstein Mini-Mental State (Folstein, Folstein, & McHugh, 1975) that required visual acuity or writing, as these were not necessary for completion of the interview. In addition, the Elderly Motivational Scale (Vallerand & O'Connor, 1991), and the Marlow-Crowne Social Desirability Scale (Strahan & Gerbasi, 1972) were all shortened, in the interest of keeping the interview as brief as possible. However, even though some measures were abbreviated, the interview was still rather lengthy. This time requirement in itself may have discouraged otherwise eligible and interested subjects from participating.

Directions for Future Research

Many of the above concerns suggest directions for potential improvement and expansion. Firstly, it would be desirable to have access to larger samples of residents, with a much higher proportion of men and person of other ethnicities included. Additionally, and as noted above, longitudinal research is necessary to track residents over time, essential to inferences regarding causality pertaining to motivational style-adjustment relationships.

REFERENCES

Abel, B., & Hayslip, B. (1986). Locus of control and adjustment to retirement. *Journal of Psychology, 120,* 479-488.

Abel, B., & Hayslip, B. (1987). Locus of control and retirement preparation. *Journal of Gerontology, 42,* 165-167.

Armer, J. M. (1996). An exploration of factors influencing adjustment among relocating rural elders. *IMAGE: Journal of Nursing Scholarship, 28,* 35-39.

Baltes, M. M. (1996). *The many faces of dependency in old age.* New York: Cambridge University Press.

Baltes, M. M., & Carstensen, L. L. (1999). Social-psychological theories and their applications to aging: From individual to collective. In V. L. Bengtson & K. W. Schaie (Eds.), *Handbook of theories of aging* (pp. 209-226). New York: Springer.

Bowsher, J. E., & Gerlach, M. J. (1990). Personal control and other determinants of psychological well-being in nursing home elders. *Scholarly Inquiry for Nursing Practice, 4,* 91-102.

Bradburn, N. M. (1969). *The structure of psychological well-being.* Chicago: Aldine.

Brandt, J., Campodonico, J. R., Rich, J. B., Baker, L., Steele, C., Ruff, T., Baker, A., & Lyketsos, C. (1998). Adjustment to residential placement in Alzheimer disease patients: Does premorbid personality matter? *International Journal of Geriatric Psychiatry, 13,* 509-515.

Claridge, K. E., Rowell, R. K., Duffy, J., & Duffy, M. (1995). Gender differences in adjustment to nursing home care. *Journal of Gerontological Social Work, 24,* 155-168.

Davidson, H. A., & O'Connor, B. P. (1990). Perceived control and acceptance of the decision to enter a nursing home as predictors of adjustment. *International Journal of Aging & Human Development, 31,* 307-318.

Fillenbaum, G. G. (1988). Multidimensional functional assessment of older adults: The duke older americans resources and services procedures. Hillsdale, NJ, England: Lawrence Erlbaum Associates, Inc.

Fleming, J. S., & Courtney, B. E. (1984). The dimensionality of self-esteem: II. Hierarchical facet model for revised measurement scales. *Journal of Personality & Social Psychology, 46,* 404-421.

Folstein, M., Anthony, J. C., Parhad, I., Duffy, B., & Gruenberg E. M. (1985). The meaning of cognitive impairment in the elderly. *Journal of the American Geriatric Society, 33,* 228-235.

Folstein, M. F., Folstein, S. E., & McHugh, P. R. (1975). Mini-mental state: A practical method for grading the cognitive status of patients for the clinician. *Journal of Psychiatric Reserves, 12,* 189-198.

Greenwood, N. A. (1999). Androgyny and adjustment in later life: Living in a veterans' home. *Journal of Clinical Geropsychology, 5,* 127-137.

Guttman, D. (1975). Parenthood: A key to the comparative study of the life cycle. In N. Datan & L. Ginsburg (Eds.), *Life-span developmental psychology: Normative life crises* (pp. 167-184). New York: Academic Press.

Hayslip, B., & Panek, P. (2002). *Adult development and aging.* Melbourne, FL: Krieger.

Hogstel, M. O. (2001). Nursing facilities. In M. O. Hogstel (Ed.), *Gerontology: Nursing care of the older adult* (pp. 387-408). Albany, NY: Delmar Publishing.

Kahn, R., & Miller, N. (1978). Assessment of altered brain function in the aged. In M. Storandt, I. Siegler, & M. Elias (Eds.), *The clinical psychology of aging* (pp. 43-69). New York: Plenum.

Katz, Downs, Cash, & Grotz. (1970); as cited in Ernst, M., & Ernst, N. S. (1984). Functional capacity. In D. J. Mangen & W. A. Peterson (Eds.), *Research Instruments in social gerontology: health, program evaluation, and demography* (pp. 9-84). Minneapolis, MN: University of Minnesota Press.

Katz, S., Ford, A. B., Moskowtiz, R. W., Jackson, B. A., & Jaffe, M. W. (1963). Studies of illness in the aged: the index of adl, a standardized measure of biological and psychological function. *Journal of the American Medical Association, 185*, 914-919.

Krichbaum, K., Ryden, M., Snyder, M., Pearson, V., Hanscom, J., Lee, H. Y., & Savik, K. (1999). The impact of transition to nursing home on elders' cognitive status, well-being, and satisfaction with nursing home. *Journal of Mental Health and Aging, 5*, 135-150.

Langley, L. K. (2001). Cognitive assessment of older adults. In R. L. Kane & R. A. Kane (Eds.), *Assessing older persons: Measures, meaning, and practical applications* (pp. 65-128). New York: Oxford.

Lohmann, N. (1977). Correlations of life satisfaction, morale, and adjustment measures. *Journal of Gerontology, 32*, 73-75.

Lorr, M., & Wunderlich, R. A. (1986). Two objective measures of self-esteem. *Journal of Personality Assessment, 50*, 18-23.

Meehan, T., Robertson, S, & Vermeer, C. (2001). The impact of relocation on elderly patients with mental illness. *Australian & New Zealand Journal of Mental Health Nursing, 10*, 236-242.

Mikhail, M. (1992). Psychological responses to relocation to a nursing home. *Journal of Gerontological Nursing, 18*, 35-39.

Moos, R. (1981). Environmental choice and control in community care settings for older people. *Journal of Applied Social Psychology, 11*, 23-43.

Moriwaki, S.Y. (1974). The Affect Balance Scale: A validity study with aged samples. *Journal of Geronotology, 29*, 73-78.

O'Connor, B. P., & Vallerand, R. J. (1994). Motivation, self-determination, and person-environment fit as predictors of psychological adjustment among nursing home residents. *Psychology and Aging, 9*, 189-194.

O'Connor, B. P., & Vallerand, R. J. (1998). Psychological adjustment variables as predictors of mortality among nursing home residents. *Psychology and Aging, 13*, 368-374.

Pearson, V. I. (2001). Assessment of function in older adults. In R. L. Kane & R. A. Kane (Eds.), *Assessing older persons: Measures, meaning, and practical applications* (pp. 17-48). New York: Oxford.

Reid, D. W., & Ziegler, M. (1981). The desired control measure and adjustment among the elderly. In H. M. Lefcourt (Ed.), *Research with the locus of control construct: Vol. 1 assessment methods.* (pp. 127-159) New York: Academic Press.

Rosenberg, M. (1965). *Society and the adolescent self-image.* Princeton, NJ: Princeton University Press.

Seligman, M. E. P. (1975). *Helplessness: On depression, development, and death.* San Franciso: W. H. Freeman.

Silber & Tippett. (1965); as cited in Blascovich, J., & Tomaka, J. (1991). Measures of self-esteem. In J. P. Robinson & P. R. Shaver (Eds), *Measures of personality and social psychological attitudes* (pp. 115-160). San Diego, CA: Academic Press, Inc.

Strahan, R., & Gerbasi, K. C. (1972). Short, homogenous versions of the marlowe-crowne social desirability scale. *Journal of Clinical Psychology, 28*, 191-193.

Tabachnick, B. G., & Fidell, L. S. (1996). *Using multivariate statistics (3rd Edition)*. New York: HarperCollins.

Vallerand, R. J., & O'Connor, B. P. (1991). Construction et validation de l'echelle de motivation pour les personnes agees (empa). [Construction and validation of the elderly motivation scale (ems)]. *International Journal of Psychology, 26*, 219-241.

Wood, V., Wylie, M. L., & Sheafor, B. (1969). An analysis of a short self-report measure of life satisfaction: correlation with rater judgments. *Journal of Gerontology, 24*, 465-469.

Ziegler, M., & Reid, D. W. (1983). Correlates of changes in desired control scores and in life satisfaction scores among elderly persons. *International Journal of Aging and Human Development, 16*, 135-145.

doi:10.1300/J137v15n04_02

The Mental Health System and Sense of Self Among Adults with Serious Mental Illness

Diane Weis Farone
Judith Pickens

SUMMARY. Development of a sense of self is a lifelong process. One's sense of continuity in the context of the demands of multiple role identities contributes to both psychological well-being and opportunities for acceptance into valued social roles. The onset of a mental illness can rupture an emerging sense of self and require intense and painful restructuring of one's beliefs and expectations. This study was a secondary analysis of qualitative data from interviews with twenty people who self-identified as having serious mental illness to explore how well the mental health system addresses the ingredients that promote, create, or restore a valued and adaptive sense of self. doi:10.1300/J137v15n04_03 *[Article copies available for a fee from The Haworth Document Delivery Service: 1-800-HAWORTH. E-mail address: <docdelivery@haworthpress.com> Website: <http://www. HaworthPress.com> © 2007 by The Haworth Press, Inc. All rights reserved.]*

KEYWORDS. Serious mental illness, identity, stigma, recovery

Diane Weis Farone, DSW, JD, is Assistant Professor, Social Work, Arizona State University at the West Campus, PO Box 37100, Phoenix, AZ 85069-7100 (E-mail: diane.farone@asu.edu). Judith Pickens, PhD, RN, is Assistant Professor, Nursing, Arizona State University at the Tempe Campus, PO Box 2602, Tempe, AZ 85287-2602 (E-mail: judith.pickens@asu.edu).

[Haworth co-indexing entry note]: "The Mental Health System and Sense of Self Among Adults with Serious Mental Illness." Farone, Diane Weis, and Judith Pickens. Co-published simultaneously in *Journal of Human Behavior in the Social Environment* (The Haworth Press, Inc.) Vol. 15, No. 4, 2007, pp. 35-54; and: *Adult Development and Well-Being: The Impact of Institutional Environments* (ed: Catherine N. Dulmus, and Karen M. Sowers) The Haworth Press, 2007, pp. 35-54. Single or multiple copies of this article are available for a fee from The Haworth Document Delivery Service [1-800-HAWORTH, 9:00 a.m. - 5:00 p.m. (EST). E-mail address: docdelivery@haworthpress.com].

INTRODUCTION

Current public policy in mental health seeks to reduce the use of hospitalization for people with serious mental illness and to develop resources that enable them to live in the community as participating and contributing members (President's New Freedom Commission on Mental Health, 2003). Within psychodynamic psychology, an experience of the self as a seamless organizer of behavior is a hallmark of well being (Mitchell & Black, 1995). Within current sociological and social psychological theory, identity as a process is what links individuals and social systems (Burke, Owens, Serpe, & Thoits, 2003). Development of a sense of who one is in relation to others begins in infancy with the establishment of core mental representations, is intensified in adolescence, and continues in dynamic interplay throughout life as new experiences and challenges are encountered.

The symptoms that define serious mental illness affect identity development in profound ways, both psychologically and socially. These symptoms often first appear in late adolescence and early adulthood, when identity development is a particular focus. The onset of a mental illness can rupture the emerging sense of self and usually requires intense and painful restructuring of one's beliefs and expectations. The central role assumed by personal identity or "sense of self" in the experience of mental illness and recovery is well-documented (Davidson & Strauss, 1992; Deegan, 1988; Estroff, 1989; Schiff, 2004; Young & Ensing, 1999). The mental health system is a community structure that is salient, for better or worse, in the negotiation of identity for those who experience the symptoms that are associated with the diagnoses that constitute serious mental illness. This paper explores how the mental health system has been experienced by a sample of twenty people with serious mental illness in ways that are relevant to the processes involved in identity development and organization of the self.

LITERATURE REVIEW

Psychological and Psychiatric Perspectives on Identity and Self

In his seminal work on identity as a developmental task, Erik Erikson (1980, p. 109) described the concept as referring to "a conscious sense of individual identity . . . an unconscious striving for a continuity of personal character . . . a criterion for the silent doings of ego synthesis, and . . .

a maintenance of an inner solidarity with a group's ideals and identity." This definition contains several functions that identity serves for both internal integrity and integration into ego syntonic, valued participation in desired social relationships.

Erikson's work started from a psychoanalytic perspective, with a model in which development is fueled by an internal thrust and molded by social experiences. What he termed identity is in many ways similar to the functions Heinz Kohut examined using the word self. Kohut also started from a psychoanalytic base in his formulation of "self psychology." Within his model (as critiqued and extensively referenced in Seigel, 1996) "narcissism," rather than Freud's libidinal drives, fuels the course of psychological development, striving towards a whole and functioning self. Kohut saw that all of us are "struggling most fundamentally with problems of self-regulation, self-esteem, and personal vitality" (Mitchell & Black, 1995, p. 165).

In Kohut's view (as summarized in Seigel, 1996), an individual develops through relationships with others. Ideally he or she has access to people who can serve as "selfobjects." A selfobject is a person who can be incorporated mentally into one's internal self structures and is, thus, accessible even when the other is not present. Selfobjects serve two necessary purposes for development of the self. One function is to provide a mirror to reflect to the individual aspects about himself or herself in a way that is experienced as an empathic understanding and acceptance. This experience of empathic acceptance allows the self to function smoothly as an integrated whole, in contrast to the unreliable performance that results from internal "splits" of one's "bad" or "unacceptable" parts, which splinters the self into non-integrated fragments.

Another type of selfobject serves as an ideal that both helps one feel safe, protected by an idealized other, and provides a model to aspire to. Internalization of the idealized selfobject gives the self system access to self management skills and principles around which to organize behavior. Failures of early relationships to provide these two "self developing" functions can give rise to distortions and defensive maneuvers. Kohut differed with traditional analysts in his definition of healthy resolution of disturbances of the self. He believed that it was not fruitful to revive narcissistic wounds from childhood, nor was a total reconstruction of the personality necessary. The self continues to seek wholeness, and current healing experiences can create compensatory structures that provide a stable, functional, and reliable self system.

Sullivan (1962) saw psychosis as existing within the context of an interpersonal field. He described the self as follows:

> There is within the personality a system of experience to which we apply the terms, the ego, or the self. This is built up of all the factors of experience that we have in which significant other people 'respond' to us. In other words, our self is made up of the reflection of our personality that we have encountered mirrored in those with whom we deal. (p. 249)

Within Sullivan's formulation anxiety has a disintegrative effect on behavioral organization. The "self" is a "gatekeeper" that attempts to ward off the experience of anxiety through mental operations. The security operations lead to defenses, distortions, and blind spots in interpersonal perception. In the extreme the distortions may be of psychotic proportions (Mitchell & Black, 1995, p. 67).

Both Sullivan and Kohut saw the resolution of dysfunctional self protective adaptations as occurring through accepting relationships. However, Sullivan described the dynamic as one of developing "social insight" to understand contexts that create the need for defensive distortions, rather than "insight into the roots of certain of his motives" (Sullivan, 1962, p. 266). Becoming symptom free would be a function of avoiding contexts that overtax one's adaptive capacities and finding or creating less dangerous or more nurturing contexts. In Kohut's model, helpful selfobject relationships are the building blocks for creating internal mental structures that create a more stable and satisfying self organization.

Sullivan's work is consistent with the work of Faris (1934) and Liang (1969) concerning problems associated with schizophrenia. Faris described the psychotic process as one in which a person must feel connected socially in order to provide a reason and means to organize his or her behavior. When excluded from social connections the person's mental experience becomes chaotic. For Liang, a weak sense of identity arises from an ontological anxiety and fear of a loss of identity through engulfment, impingement, or depersonalization. Health is described as an ontological security, in which one can "encounter all the hazards of life, social, ethical, spiritual, biological, from a centrally firm sense of his own and the other people's reality and identity" (Liang, p. 39). This description bears a resemblance to Kohut's description of a smoothly functioning self system.

Sociological Perspectives on Identity

Within the tradition of symbolic interactionism (Cooley, 1902; Mead, 1934) we learn who we are by seeing ourselves through the eyes of others. The ability to take the perspective of others is what enables us to discern norms and role expectations. Participation in social roles provides meaning to individual lives and continuity and purpose in functioning for the society. Because we occupy multiple roles, we adopt various identities according to the expectations associated with the different relationships in which we are involved. Because we seek approval, we try to comport our behavior in accordance with what we perceive to be the social norms. It is through this mechanism that society is replicated over time.

In an attempt to synthesize the idea of identity as a social product with the idea of identity as a social force, Hunt (2003, p. 71) described identities as "internalized self-designations based on the meanings (role expectations) attached to positions in social structure (role involvements)." Identities are a product of the meanings and expectations, and the individual participates as an agent in negotiating the requirements of his or her participation. In Hunt's view identities are multiple, based in the various roles occupied by the self, which positions are "organized into a saliency hierarchy" (Hunt, 2003, p. 72).

Thoits (1985, 2003) has explored the value of multiple identities as a buffer against psychological distress within the general population. According to Thoits (2003), role participation provides a sense of purpose and meaning in life and guidance for behavior, which reduces depression and anxiety. Also, successful role performance enhances self efficacy. Thoits' work supports the idea that participating in more roles provides a richer, more creative life, when the additional roles are voluntarily entered into. Obligatory roles, such as those associated with being a family member, often contain conflicts that counterbalance the roles' potential as supportive and enriching resources, making their effects on psychological well-being more ambiguous or problematic (Lincoln, 2000; Rosenfield & Wenzel, 1997).

Also within the tradition of symbolic interactionism, and more germane to people with psychiatric diagnoses is Goffman's (1963) work regarding stigma and labeling. Within this view, normal development of one's identity comes about through an ability to see ourselves as we think others see us and to compare how we see ourselves with what we perceive as being valued by our social groups. For whatever reasons, there are attributes that are, or become, "stigmatized" by social groups (see also Foucault, 1976). Having one or more of those attributes exposes one to the risk of being "discredited" if the attribute is known or "discreditable" if it is not known. This situation presents the bearer of the attribute with several challenges: to internalize or deconstruct the meaning of the stigma, to disclose or not disclose the attribute (in cases, such as mental illness, where it may not be readily observable), to choose whether or when to align oneself with the dominant ("normal") or non-dominant (stigmatized) group, and to generally manage one's day to day life, relationships, and sense of self esteem or self efficacy. Stigma has been identified by both the mental health system (U.S. Department of Health and Human Services, 1999), people with psychiatric diagnoses (DeNiro, 1995; Onken, Dumont, Ridgway, Dornan, & Ralph, 2002; Wahl, 1999), and researchers (Link, 1987; Link, Cullen, Struening, Shrout, & Dohrenwend, 1989) alike as a major challenge for recovery, sometimes more difficult than management of the symptoms of the disorder.

Wolfensberger (1972, 1999, 2000) has conceptualized an ethical and appropriate human services response to stigmatized identities through policies of normalization and social role valorization. His work grew from concern for people with developmental disabilities (mental retardation), and has been applied in the mental health field (Flynn & Aubry, 1999; Reidy, 1999). Normalization refers to policies that support enabling people with disabilities to live a life that is as close to normal as possible (Wolfensberger, 1972, p. 27). Social role valorization refers to increasing the value attached to varied social roles or creating new roles that are less devalued than those generally available to people with stigmatized statuses, such as "mental patient." The intent of normalization and social role valorization is to facilitate participation by people with disabilities in meaningful, valued ways in the community. In service of being realistic, Wolfensberger cautions that "social and societal devaluation is a universal; . . . that all social systems have a limit to their capacity to assimilate dissimilar people; . . . and that one cannot bludgeon humans into liking others, being good to them, and wanting them around" (Wolfensberger, 1999, p. 494). Nevertheless, Reidy (1999) argues that a recovery philosophy requires human service personnel to work for greater accommodations on the part of communities to make room for people with diverse abilities to thrive.

In summary, a stable and integrated sense of self is an important component of both psychological well-being and opportunities for full participation in valued social roles. Access to valued social roles is, in turn, related to well-being and to inclusion into meaningful lives in the community. The theoretical models of Sullivan, Faris, Kohut, and Liang suggest that a major task of recovery is to bolster a sense of self in all aspects of the word–continuity of individual existence, personal agency, and solidarity with some social group. Important ingredients would be those that enhance self regulation of emotional distress, stimulate motivation to risk entering into relationships, foster insight into characteristics of different social contexts, and provide recognition and acceptance. Institutional services should offer support, encouragement, and a sounding board that can help people sort through their thoughts, feelings, and aspirations; make decisions; and sustain the courage and efforts required to consolidate a functional and stable "self" connection. Sociological concepts of "the looking glass self" (Cooley, 1902) and "spoiled identities" (Goffman, 1963) also point to the importance of building role taking skills and creating an accepting and valuing social context, at best, or at least a facilitation of the deconstruction of internalized stigma. The question asked of the data, then, was, "to what extent, and in what ways, does the mental health system address the ingredients that promote, create, or restore a valued and adaptive sense of self?"

METHODOLOGY

This paper is based on an analysis of descriptions by people with serious mental illness of their experiences with components of the mental health system. This is a secondary analysis of data originally collected to explore the circumstances under which people with serious mental illness experience a sense of belonging.

The study included a convenience sample of twenty people from the community who volunteered to participate. The procedures for recruitment, interviewing, and maintaining confidentiality were approved by the Institutional Review Board for the university with which the investigators are associated. Each investigator interviewed ten people who identified themselves as having a serious mental illness. Two subsequent focus groups were conducted to follow up on some of the themes that had been identified from the initial individual interviews. Except for two members of one group, the focus groups consisted of people who had already been interviewed individually. All interviews were professionally transcribed and then evaluated separately by each investigator. The two investigators met periodically to discuss their identification of themes and to reach consensus.

The study sample consisted of nine males and 11 females. The mean age was 47 and the range was from 18 to 60. Eight were interviewed at a consumer-run drop-in center, four at a consumer-run rehabilitation center, six in their group homes, and two at public community locations. Diagnoses, identified by self report, included bipolar disorder (5), major depression (6), schizophrenic disorders (6), dissociative identity disorder (1), post traumatic stress disorder (1), and attention deficit hyperactivity disorder (1, an 18 year old male).

FINDINGS

One striking feature of the study was the infrequency of references to the formal mental health system as a place associated with belonging. The importance of peer-run drop-in centers and wellness programs provided a strong contrast, offering an important space for developing a clearer and more accepting sense of self.

When mentioned at all as a positive, the formal system was seen as helpful in providing information and assistance with concrete needs, especially housing. The system's role in relation to housing was not always positive, however, due to long waiting lists and frequent relocations. To a male participant from a drop-in center, the provision of housing by his case manager was a turning point in his road to recovery:

> I think that that was a time when I started to go so far into the pit that there was no way I was to turn but to go up. I mean I was close to death and I didn't care . . . Somehow, somewhere [my case manager] got me my housing and that's when things started to turn around for me . . . Being homeless . . . I'd go into depression real fast, real quick, but then [my case manager] helped me out with my housing and they're still going to send me to school for computer repair. I screwed that up by drinking too much. I told my voc rehab counselor I want to get some real sobriety time under my belt before I decide to go back . . . I don't want to screw it up. It is a $15,000 education being given to me for free.

In a focus group discussion about what the mental health system should be providing, another male participant from a drop-in center immediately responded:

A lot more housing. They should have a time limit on waiting lists so 3 or 4 years don't go by before you can get in it . . . I'm homeless now, and its bothering me mentally, you know, 'cause I'm hearing a lot of voices and all the people are talking . . . I stay in the shelter sometimes. The shelter costs us two to three dollars a night. That's hard to get up sometimes . . . It's cold at night. I ain't slept none last night so I am really a long ways from being myself.

A third perspective on the part housing plays in establishing oneself in the community is the issue of being moved from one place to another. As a male participant from a group home said:

You can't give a mentally ill person a feeling of security in their own home where they are living or residing if you keep moving them every 6 months to a year to a year and a half like [my provider] does with their program system of 24, 16, 8 hours. You can't give them a feeling of security ever. They will constantly be in a state of mental disruption . . . A sense of security is impossible the way [my provider] is running this system, . . . [as are a sense] of feeling like you're safe, of feeling like you ever could belong to a structure that you could call home.

For one young man in a group home, aging out of the juvenile system into the adult system precipitated a wrenching separation from an attachment he had formed in a former group home. Two participants, one male and one female, who were living in a group home felt alienated because they felt they were of a higher functional level than the other residents in their respective group homes. Another male who had moved from a group home to an individual apartment was glad he no longer had roommates, and a female who had been moved from an individual apartment back to a group home due to budget cuts described her roommate as "depressing" to be around.

Apparent in these experiences is the significance of housing. A home should provide the shelter and safety necessary to free one to pursue longer term aspects of recovery. As can be seen in the participants' comments, the kind of housing solution also affects multiple aspects concerning one's identity and sense of self. Frequency of moves interrupts continuity of existence. When moves and roommates are determined by the mental health system, a sense of agency is undermined. Identifying housing arrangements according to level of care may be designed to match need with resources and to motivate people to seek higher functional levels. However, such classifications also label a person in ways that are socially apparent and are often experienced as stigmatizing.

A second theme that was expressed by a majority of the twenty interviewees was the importance of feeling accepted. They overwhelmingly endorsed consumer run settings as places that were safe, comfortable, and non-judgmental. Safety meant it is not necessary to worry about maintaining secrecy, nor does one have to worry about being rejected for having a "bad day" or appearance of symptoms. As one female employee of a consumer run agency put it:

> I have always had trouble holding–well, not holding–but being accepted at a job, other than here with other people who are mentally ill. I can hold a job. It's just harder. They do not recognize the symptoms. If I need a time out away from, or an extra break I can get it here. They are not willing to do that on normal jobs.

A male attendee of a consumer drop-in center said:

> You know, people here, they, no one is trying to impress you with their intellectual ability, their knowledge, or anything like that. You know, everyone just comes here and it's kind of common knowledge that each one has a mental illness of some type. And, I guess that's why people get along so well, because if someone starts acting, you know, odd, with odd behavior, you know, they might be going through a rough time.

Another male attendee of the center provided a detailed description of its meanings to him:

> I feel accepted here . . . It's a place where I could just walk in the front door and grab a cup of coffee and not have to worry about being judged . . . [At first] I came for the food, to tell you the truth . . . But, I started learning about the other programs that they got . . . And it was a place for me to get out of my house, get out of my own mind for a while, sit back and relax . . . It's a safe sober environment and I like it like that . . . I feel an obligation to this place, actually, because they have given a lot to me. They have given me peace of mind, they've given me clothes, they've helped me when I am feeling so down that I have no where else to turn . . . It is

like a refuge for me . . . When they put me behind the desk [as a receptionist] and got me running groups and stuff, I like to go home feeling that I have actually helped some people over here, which makes me feel good about myself.

The ingredients of acceptance, valued roles, and opportunities for multiple roles are all apparent in the above passage. The same participant also reflected on the value of an "idealized" role model. In describing how he learned to cope with a problem that arose when he was manning the reception desk, he said, "[One of the paid consumer staff members] has been one of the greatest teachers I have studied under. I watch her and she's got a real easy going attitude. I try to handle things the way she would."

These observations about peer run organizations provide a sharp contrast to the following comments about the formal system providers, beginning with a female employee of a consumer run agency in one of the focus groups, who contrasts the two:

My original answer when I went through this was the people that I felt I connected the most with were other people with serious mental illness. I felt there was no need to explain anything. There was acceptan . . . ce[I can connect] when I'm in a place where I don't have to worry about the stigma, or that my thoughts will be judged, or anyone will treat me differently because of it. Where it is safe to say, the most bizarre is where I can connect. I cannot say these things to [my provider agency] . . . It's almost like the system itself is an unsafe place. Wait till you tell the system. They give you another label and, by god, you must have another drug . . . Maybe they didn't need the drug in the first place. Maybe they just needed someone to listen and not drugs . . . They [the system] can't hear it. That's why this peer stuff works and that's why I can connect, because I don't have to be afraid that a peer, someone who also has a label, is going to judge me, label me, or call the crisis line on me, or try to talk me into going into the hospital and give me an antipsychotic drug . . . It's almost like the system itself is so unsafe to even talk about. So the only place I really connect well is in the waiting room with someone else that is not afraid to talk to me. When we folks get out here and nobody else is listening, we do help quite nicely with each other.

Some specific examples of experiences of the formal system as unsafe include:

> As far as feeling disrespected, is usually when I go to [my provider agency] and it's kind of like some of the things they tell you insults your intelligence. There have been a couple of occasions when I've had to tell some of my case managers, look, you need to not talk to me in this manner, you know. I am just as well educated or more so than you are and you need to talk to me at a level such as that, not like I'm a little child that, you know, you have to pacify or you have to just tell me what I want to hear, knowing that it's not going to ever come about. (Male at a drop-in center)
>
> I made the mistake of taking some of my poems in to a psychiatrist that hadn't been exposed to poetry because I mentioned . . . that writing was therapeutic for me and sometimes other people got a charge out of it too . . . She said, ok, well bring one in. So I brought one in. And I found out later that what had gone on my record was, ah, life of fantasy and delusions and clanging behavior. They even have a word for the symptom, clanging behavior. People who compulsively talk in rhymes. So that was the last time I talked about my poetry to the system. (Male from the community, whose poetry has been published)
>
> I was born . . . in a large Catholic family and we talked fast. It was always just a joke ... how I was taught to speak to a phonograph designed–and if you are old enough to understand this–to a record that was supposed to play at 33 1/3 that was played at 78 . . . Once I got a label [diagnosis], and I got access to some of my records . . . I was in there always diagnosed with pressured speech. (Female employee of consumer run agency)

These examples poignantly illustrate the experience of invalidation through language and social process. The labels lead to one or more of several resolutions–alienation from oneself, self doubt and inner conflict, social withdrawal, or social action to advocate for change. The following are some eloquent words to describe recovery through the eyes of the study participants:

> I feel valued when I am employed; when my medication is stable; when I'm accepted–when I do self talk with my self esteem to keep it above water . . . The tools that they gave me through the WRAP

[Wellness Recovery Action Plan] book really helped me. Which was finding out, you know, what makes me, what triggers me, what makes me feel like that, what I can do about it to get my connection back. (Female peer run agency employee)

I am not as needy of others' validation as I used to be in life because of how I felt. Because of not knowing who I was–forgetting who I was because of the experiences . . . When I began to think about that and journal about that and pray about that, I discovered that I could actually remember who I was before the incident occurred . . . That is how I knew that I got lost in the shuffle somewhere . . . It wasn't until certain things went into place when I couldn't function any more and found myself with a full blown diagnosis besides behaviors that I got totally lost. All I knew was who I was in relation to my roles in life. And, judged myself into what I did. And then getting back into finding out who I was got me into remembering the gifts that I was born with . . . In discovering that I was whole and complete has helped me feel more comfortable and connected to non-diagnosed people. (Female peer run agency employee)

This same individual went on to say that when she was diagnosed her life was all illness. When she discovered recovery, her life was all recovery. When she got spirituality, recovery remained as a small portion of her life, but most of it was about life, by which she meant, "I feel like a human being fulfilling a purpose and having a meaning in life."

A female resident of a group home had a profound vision of her aspirations, but had not reached them:

I got it [schizophrenia]. It's better though. My medications are helping me . . . About belonging. I won't feel belonging, I guess, until I get on my own . . . I always felt alone, like an outcast and different from my family . . . Maybe I don't know what belonging means. I always thought belonging means you fit in, you know, I guess I don't have that . . . I would like to have friends I want to talk to and go places and do things . . . I want to go freely, you know and have my own place, and don't have roommates and authority figures over me all the time telling me what to do, how to do it. One of my goals is to be medication free . . . I want my independence and I don't want like the government and them people in my business. I don't want to be in the system . . . I just don't want to have no diagnosis.

DISCUSSION

Multiple theorists have conceptualized a psychological mechanism that regulates mental processes internally and adapts behavior to the requirements and opportunities contained in environmental contexts. The mechanism is a process that continues to evolve throughout life, and one that is responsive to both internal and external stimulation. The elements that support what Karl Menninger (1963) referred to as the "vital balance" that characterizes mental and emotional well-being include basic health and nutrition, some predictability and control of environmental demands for adaptation, empathic validation of one's being, and successes that build feelings of self efficacy.

What does the mental health system as an institution contribute to ongoing self development for people with serious mental illnesses? Onken et al. (2002) in summarizing the findings from multiple representative focus groups of people from nine states who have major psychiatric diagnoses characterized some of the issues as follows:

> We must fully acknowledge that the formal system often hinders recovery through bureaucratic program guidelines, limited access to services and supports, abusive practices, poor quality services, negative messages, lack of 'best practice' program elements, and a narrow focus on a bio-psychiatric orientation that can actually serve to discount the person's humanity . . . At the core of such hindering forces is the operationalization of society's response to mental illness, that of shame and hopelessness and the need to assert social control over the unknown and uncomfortable. (p. ix)

Inclusion of case management to create linkages with needed basic services such as housing, income, and appropriate job placement are conceptually an integral part of best practices for community mental health efforts. Spontaneous reflections of our study participants testify to the importance of stability and continuity in getting basic needs met in order to undertake the work of recovery. Several study participants acknowledged that their case managers were helpful in this regard. Findings from the many studies of assertive community treatment and intensive case management services indicate that these services are valuable even beyond the material benefits they provide. Facilitating access to resources that meet basic needs enhances engagement with the helping process and is associated with more favorable outcomes in terms of symptom reduction and social functioning (Chinman, Allende, Bailey, Maust, & Davidson, 1999; Ziguras & Stuart, 2000).

On the other hand, when obtaining access to resources seems to recipients to be tied to acceptance of a label of mental illness, or to require "compliant behavior" in order not to be "cut off," engagement that is constructive to positive self development may be impaired. The person may feel more vulnerable and/or more controlled or coerced.

Many of the study participants' comments emphasize the importance of agency and choice, a finding consistent with those of other qualitative studies involving people with serious mental illnesses (Barry, Zeber, Blow, & Valenstein, 2003; Davidson, 2003). Opportunities for choice and agency can be experienced within the mental health system. Only one participant talked specifically about the coercive power of the system, and he was the only interviewee who was at the time under court mandated treatment. However, other studies have found more subtle interactions with providers are experienced as coercive and lead to a disengagement from, or failure to establish engagement with, the service system (Watts & Priebe, 2002). Several study participants mentioned feeling unsafe from invalidation, paternalistic responses, and prescription of unwanted medications. Disengagement and defensive secrecy can operate to block access to services that could be helpful.

Structurally the mental health system has substantial power. It is responsible for treating a broad spectrum of disorders and is held accountable by third parties for protection against danger to self or others and is expected to reduce symptoms and improve social functioning. Being held to such standards creates a pressure to control and increases the risk of underestimating the capacities of people in order to avoid the risk of "bad" results. Hierarchical exercise of authority affects both disempowerment of agency and damage to self validation through stigma. A growing emphasis on consumerism and the recovery model is challenging the mental health system to release some control. Doing so tends to raise many questions. Would there be a negative impact on the prevalence of behaviors that are dangerous for self or others? Does release of control and encouraging empowerment reduce symptoms and facility utilization? Would or should there be modifications in legal standards and funders' expectations of the system? Do conceptualizations about what is defined as dysfunctional need to be deconstructed and reconstructed? Would some release of control reflect or lead to a reduction in the degree of stigma associated with the mental health system because of its historical coercive role?

Pinfold (2000), in an attempt to summarize issues surrounding community mental health policies, aptly pointed out that:

> While discussions on how to improve community mental health care systems continue, people who suffer mental health problems are having to cope with their illness in a society that, in the main, retains distance between the self and those perceived as 'other.' (p. 202)

The association between a pathology orientation and stigma, whether in the eyes of the potential consumer or the general public or both, is an aspect of the medical model that is challenging to actual and potential users of the mental health system (Link, 1987; Link et al., 1989; Pescosolido, Monahan, Lind, Stueve, & Kikuzawa, 1999). The issue of stigma is a conundrum for the system. Becoming a part of the mental health system is often experienced as an internalization of a stigmatized label and a further devaluation of the self. This presents a dilemma that is common in many fields of human service. Creating categories recognizes social problems and suggests steps needed to address them, but the creation of the category has the unintended consequence of stigmatizing the intended beneficiaries of the services.

To totally deconstruct the concept of mental illness would leave many without essential services. To retain the categories contributes to the experience of stigma. The reconstruction of mental illness as a "brain disease" rather than a mental or psychological disease appears to alleviate internalized stigma somewhat (Mechanic, McAlpine, Rosenfield, & Davis, 1999). Goffman, Foucault, and Wolfensberger suggest that stigma needs to be deconstructed and more opportunities for participation in valued social roles need to be developed. Attention to stigma and social stratification inherent in being a part of the mental health system is readily apparent in this study, again a finding that is consistent with previous research (DeNiro, 1995; Link, 1987; Link et al., 1989; Wahl, 1999). The system cannot eliminate the human tendency to create social stratifications, which is even practiced by some people with psychiatric diagnoses among themselves. However, peer run organizations and groups seems to be playing an important role in the deconstruction and restructuring of concepts related to mental illness and stigma.

Trust and constructive engagement with the system grow from one's sense of being accepted and perception of a desire on the part of the provider to work collaboratively. In a study comparing results for men in the VA system who had psychotic diagnoses and histories of 150 days or more of psychiatric hospitalization who received assertive community treatment (ACT) with those who participated in a strengths based program, those in the strengths based program showed significantly more improvement in the reduction of both positive and negative symptoms (Barry et al., 2003). The two major differences between the two models were the strengths based emphasis on relationship to an individual, rather than to the team, and its emphasis on strengths rather than pathologies or problems. The findings suggest that symptoms may serve as an adaptive solution to excess stress and that acceptance, valuation, and greater freedom to be "who one is" reduces the need for symptoms and releases a smoother self regulation process.

In summary, based on the participants' descriptions, the mental health system is valued as a source of information, concrete assistance, and medication that relieves some symptoms. Although participants may not be aware of it, the system also finances the peer run resources they so strongly endorse. The medical model, with its role as expert, its application of labels, and its structures for efficiency and objectivity is experienced at best as neutral and often as negative. A hope that is reflected in the public policy to support consumer participation in mental health services planning and delivery at all levels is that the system will become more collaborative. A hope inherent in the idea of recovery is that more people with serious mental illness will feel empowered to find social interaction, social acceptance, social support, and meaningful participation in the general community. They will, thus, be less stigmatized for at least two reasons. One is that their participation is not defined by their mental illness. The other is that the way public prejudices are changed is through close association with a person who has the stigmatized condition. That kind of association allows for knowing the person as a whole human being, rather than as a particular attribute (Clinton, 1999; Corrigan, Lundin, Kubiak, & Penn, 2001; Davidson, Stayner, Nickou, Styron, Rowe, & Chinman, 2001; Kolodziej & Johnson, 1996).

REFERENCES

Barry, K.L., Zeber, J.E., Blow, F.C., & Valenstein, M. (2003). Effect of strengths model versus assertive community treatment model on participant outcomes and utilization: Two-Year follow-up. *Psychiatric Rehabilitation Journal, 26,* 268-277.

Burke, P.J., Owens, T.J., Serpe, R.T., & Thoits, P.A. (Eds.). (2003). *Advances in identity theory and research.* New York: Kluwer Academic/Plenum Publishers.

Chinman, M., Allende, M., Bailey, P., Maust, J., & Davidson, L. (1999). Therapeutic agents of assertive community treatment. *Psychiatric Quarterly, 70,* 137-162.

Clinton, M. (1999). Collaborative education and social stereotypes. *Australian and New Zealand Journal of Mental Health Nursing, 8,* 100-103.
Cooley, C.H. (1902). *Human nature and social order.* New York: Scribners.
Corrigan, P.W., Green, A., Lundin, R., Kubiak, M.A., & Penn, L. (2001). Familiarity with and social distance from people who have serious mental illness. *Psychiatric Services, 52,* 953-958.
Davidson, L. (2003). *Living outside mental illness: Qualitative studies of recovery in schizophrenia.* New York: New York University Press.
Davidson, L., Stayner, D.A., Nickou, C., Styron, T.H., Rowe, M., & Chinman, M.L. (2001). Simply to be let in: Inclusion as a basis for recovery. *Psychiatric Rehabilitation Journal, 24,* 375-388.
Davidson, L., & Strauss, J.S. (1992). Sense of self in recovery from severe mental illness. *British Journal of Medical Psychology, 65,* 131-145.
Deegan, P.E. (1988). Recovery: The lived experience of rehabilitation. *Psychosocial Rehabilitation Journal, 11,* 11-19.
DeNiro, D.A. (1995). Perceived alienation in individuals with residual-type schizophrenia. *Issues in Mental Health Nursing, 16,* 185-200.
Erikson, E.H. (1980). *Identity and the life cycle.* New York: W.W. Norton & Company.
Estroff, S.E. (1989). Self, identity, and subjective experiences of schizophrenia: In search of the subject. *Schizophrenia Bulletin, 15,* 189-196.
Faris, R.E. (1934). Cultural isolation and the schizophrenic personality. *American Journal of Sociology, 40,* 155-169.
Flynn, R.J., & Aubry, T.D. (1999). Integration of persons with developmental or psychiatric disabilities: Conceptualization and measurement. In R.J. Flynn & R.A. Lemay (Eds.), *A Quarter-century of Normalization and Social Role Valorization: Evolution and Impact* (pp. 271-303). Ottawa: University of Ottawa Press.
Foucault, M. (1954). *Mental illness and psychology.* Berkeley, CA: University of California Press.
Goffman, E. (1963). *Stigma: Notes on the management of spoiled identity.* New York: Simon & Schuster, Inc.
Hunt, M.O. (2003). Identity and inequality: Exploring links between self and stratification processes. In P.J. Burke, T.J. Owens, R.T. Serpe, & P.A. Thoits (Eds.), *Advances in identity theory and research* (pp. 71-84). New York: Kluwer Academic/ Plenum Publishers.
Kolodziej, M., & Johnson, B.T. (1996). Interpersonal contact and acceptance of persons with psychiatric disorders: A research synthesis. *Journal of Consulting and Clinical Psychology, 64,* 1387-1396.
Liang, R.D. (1969). *The Divided self.* London: Penguin Books, Ltd.
Lincoln, K.D. (2000). Social support, negative social interactions, and psychological well-being. *Social Service Review, 74,* 231-252.
Link, B.G. (1987). Understanding labeling effects in the area of mental disorders: An assessment of the effects of expectations of rejection. *American Sociological Review, 52,* 96-112.
Link, B.G., Cullen, F.T., Struening, E., Shrout, P.E., & Dohrenwend, B.P. (1989). A modified labeling theory approach to mental disorder: An empirical assessment. *American Sociological Review, 54,* 400-423.

Mead, G.H. (1934). *Mind, self, and society.* Chicago: University of Chicago Press.
Mechanic, D., McAlpine, D., Rosenfield, S., & Davis, D. (1994). Effects of illness attribution and depression on the quality of life among persons with serious mental illness. *Social Science Medicine, 39,* 155-164.
Menninger, K. (1963). *The vital balance.* New York: Viking Press.
Mitchell, S.A., & Black, M.J. (1995). *Freud and beyond: A history of modern psycho-analytic thought.* New York: Basic Books.
Onken, S.J., Dumont, J.M., Ridgway, P., Dornan, D.H., & Ralph, R.O. (October, 2002). Mental health recovery: What helps and what hinders? Alexandria, VA: National Technical Assistance Center for State Mental Health Planning. Retrieved July18, 2003, FROM www.nasmhpd.org/ntac/reports/MHSIPReport.pdf.
Pescosolido, B.A., Monahan, J., Link, B.G., Stueve, A., & Kiduzawa, S. (1999). The public's view of the competence, dangerousness, and need for legal coercion of persons with mental health problems. *American Journal of Public Health, 89,* 1339-1345.
Pinfold, V. (2000). 'Building up safe havens...all around the world': Users' experiences of living in the community with mental health problems. *Health & Place, 6,* 201-212.
President's New Freedom Commission on Mental Health. (2003). Achieving the promise: Transforming mental health care in America. Washington, DC: Department of Health and Human Services Publication No. SMA-03-3832.
Reidy, D. (1999). Social integration: How can we get there from here? Reflections on normalization, social role valorization and community education. In R.J. Flynn & R.A. Lemay (Eds.), *A Quarter-Century of Normalization and Social Role Valorization: Evolution and Impact* (pp. 375-384). Ottawa: University of Ottawa Press.
Rosenfield, S., & Wenzel, S. (1997). Social networks and chronic mental illness: A test of four perspectives. *Social Problems, 44,* 200-216.
Schiff, A.C. (2004). Recovery and mental illness: Analysis and personal reflections. *Psychiatric Rehabilitation Journal, 27,* 212-218.
Seigel, A.M. (1996). *Heinz Kohut and the psychology of the self.* Philadelphia: Brunner-Routledge.
Sullivan, H.S. (1962). *Schizophrenia as a human process.* New York: W.W. Norton & Company, Inc.
Thoits, P.A. (1985). Self-labeling processes in mental illness: The role of emotional deviance. *American Journal of Sociology, 91,* 221-249.
Thoits, P.A. (2003). Personal agency in the accumulation of multiple role-identities. In P.J. Burke, T.J. Owens, R.T. Serpe, & P.A. Thoits (Eds.), *Advances in identity theory and research* (pp. 179-194). New York: Kluwer Academic/Plenum Publishers.
U.S. Department of Health and Human Services (1999). Mental health: A report of the surgeon general. Rockville, MD: U.S. Department of Health and Human Services, Substance Abuse and Mental Health Services Administration, Center for Mental Health Services, National Institute of Health, National Institute of Mental Health.
Wahl, O.F. (1999). Mental health consumers' experience of stigma. *Schizophrenia Bulletin, 25,* 467-478.
Watts, J., & Priebe, S. (2002). A phenomenological account of users' experiences of assertive community treatment. *Bioethics, 16,* 439-454.

Wolfensberger, W. (1972). *Normalization: The principle of normalization in human services.* Toronto: National Institute on Mental Retardation.
Wolfensberger, W. (1999). Concluding reflections and a look ahead into the future for normalization and social role valorization. In R.J. Flynn & R.A. Lemay (Eds.), *A Quarter-Century of normalization and social role valorization: Evolution and impact* (pp. 489-504). Ottawa: University of Ottawa Press.
Wolfensberger, W. (2000). A brief overview of social role valorization. *Mental Retardation, 38,* 105-123.
Young, S., & Ensing, D. (1999). Exploring recovery from the perspective of people with psychiatric disabilities. *Psychiatric Rehabilitation Journal, 22,* 219-231.
Ziguras, S.J., & Stuart, G.W. (2000). A meta-analysis of the effectiveness of mental health case management over 20 years. *Psychiatric Services, 51,* 1410-1421.

doi:10.1300/J137v15n04_03

Caregiving and Welfare Reform:
Voices of Low-Income Foster Mothers

Filomena M. Critelli

SUMMARY. Welfare reform policies instituted in 1996 have significantly altered the context in which care is performed by diminishing resources available to poor mothers and places further limits on full-time caregiving as an option for them. This has created additional challenges for low-income foster mothers, many of whom are women of color. Based upon interviews in English and Spanish with 100 foster mothers on TANF, this study explores care-giving as an important aspect of gender and cultural identity and survival strategy for these foster mothers. The perceptions and experiences of poor women caring for troubled children with limited resources are viewed in the context of welfare reform. Policy considerations regarding caregiving are also discussed. doi:10.1300/J137v15n04_04 *[Article copies available for a fee from The Haworth Document Delivery Service: 1-800-HAWORTH. E-mail address: <docdelivery@haworthpress.com> Website: <http://www. HaworthPress.com> © 2007 by The Haworth Press, Inc. All rights reserved.]*

KEYWORDS. Welfare reform, caregiving, foster mothers

Filomena M. Critelli, PhD, LCSW, is affiliated with University of Buffalo School of Social Work, 665 Baldy Hall, Buffalo, NY 14260 (E-mail: fmc8@buffalo.edu).

[Haworth co-indexing entry note]: "Caregiving and Welfare Reform: Voices of Low-Income Foster Mothers." Critelli, Filomena M. Co-published simultaneously in *Journal of Human Behavior in the Social Environment* (The Haworth Press, Inc.) Vol. 15, No. 4, 2007, pp. 55-80; and: *Adult Development and Well-Being: The Impact of Institutional Environments* (ed: Catherine N. Dulmus, and Karen M. Sowers) The Haworth Press, 2007, pp. 55-80. Single or multiple copies of this article are available for a fee from The Haworth Document Delivery Service [1-800-HAWORTH, 9:00 a.m. - 5:00 p.m. (EST). E-mail address: docdelivery@haworthpress.com].

INTRODUCTION

The vast changes in the U.S. welfare system ushered in by the Personal Responsibility and Work Opportunity Reconciliation Act (PRWORA) of 1996 signify a 180-degree shift in the policy pendulum from the intentions expressed in the Social Security Act that sought to enable women to remain at home to care for their children. Current U.S. welfare policy has dramatically altered the context in which care is performed by diminishing resources available to poor mothers and placing further limits full-time caregiving as an option for them (Michel, 2000; Oliker, 2000; Mink, 1998, 1999).

Work-first policies and "get tough" practices designed to reduce the problem of "welfare dependency" are moving women from welfare into the workforce. While officials may boast of the tremendous reduction of the welfare caseloads, other potential social costs were not calculated in the drafting of the legislation. The resulting reduction of state services and push toward female employment creates a greater burden for women and in many cases a reduction of caregiving (George and Wilding, 2002). Poorer families, especially women of color who are parenting alone and whose prospects in the labor market often do not entail earning living wages cannot afford to make up the deficit in care by paying for private services to carry out domestic and caring roles. One key population of women whose needs were not considered in this legislation are low-income mothers who receive TANF to care for their birth children while caring for foster children for the child welfare system.

Challenging the Stereotype–Foster Mothers on Welfare

The term "welfare mother" conjures up images of irresponsible, lazy, sexually promiscuous, immoral women who are constructed as nonproductive, even bad mothers. These stereotypes diminish and obscure the mothering aspect of the term and the difficulties of providing care to children in conditions of poverty.

There is probably no group that embodies contradictions in current public policy in the United States than low-income foster mothers who are also TANF recipients. Several years after the implementation of welfare reform, it was estimated that as many as 40% to 60% of foster parents were receiving public assistance in New York City and providing care to society's most needy children (Fifield and Helper, 1999; Zimmerman et al., 1998; The Administration for Children's Services, 1997). Many are kinship foster mothers who are providing continuity and stability to relatives' children who would otherwise be placed with strangers (U.S. GAO 1999; Goerge, 1999; Gleeson, 1996; Dubowitz et al., 1993; Berrick et al., 1994; Hegar and Scannapieco, 1995). The interlocking oppressions of race, gender, ethnicity and class are fully represented in the foster mother population, who in large cities such New York City are primarily low-income women of color (Zimmerman et al., 1998).

A sound analysis of policies affecting women must recognize inequalities among women and assess their impact on differently situated women (Mink, 2001). State welfare policies often reinforce gender, class and race/ethnic disparities in societies through shrinking entitlements to the poor and inattention to how the work of reproduction gets done (Gordon, 1990; Abramovitz, 1988; Sainsbury, 1999; Michel, 2000; Oliker, 2000). How states treat the work involved in reproduction, together with whom they entitle and to what, is therefore crucially important to women's well-being and the availability of options (Meyer, 2000; Oliker, 2000; Sen, 1994).

The policy changes of welfare reform devalues of mothering of all poor women, but are all the more striking when considering foster mothers, who provide a valuable service by caring for children in state custody. Foster mothers' care-giving responsibilities result in personal and economic costs for them. Welfare reform has removed access to income support that enabled them to provide foster care services requiring that they combine work with their fostering responsibilities. Foster mothers are subject to the five-year time limit under TANF and are not eligible for federally funded benefits after that time.

Brief Historical Background

Gender and racial inequalities have been reflected in welfare programs since their inception (Gordon, 1994). The traditional division of labor between men as earners and women as caregivers produces a gender differentiation of social rights and benefit levels so that formal employment has resulted in better welfare state entitlements than informal caring (Abramovitz, 1988; Miller, 1990; Gordon, 1990; Sainsbury, 1996; and Mink, 1999). Nevertheless, concern for single mothers and their children were a major influence on the development of modern welfare policy, with the goal of relieving poor single mothers of the necessity of wage earning so that they might care full-time for their children (Abramovitz, 1988; Miller, 1990). The early Mother's Pensions were designed as a payment for the services of motherhood, although they almost exclusively served white widows (Gordon, 1990).

Aid to Dependent Children (ADC) was created in 1935 as a critical piece of legislation during the New Deal and recipients were expanded to include mothers who were abandoned, divorced, never married, or mothers whose husbands were unable to work (Gordon, 1990; Quadagno, 1994). In the wake of social policy changes of the 1960s and 1970s, as eligibility barriers to AFDC fell, increasing proportions of the single mothers depending on AFDC were women of color, due to demographic differences and their greater vulnerability to poverty (Quadagno, 1994; Seccombe, 1999).

Within the child welfare system, this lead to an increased reliance on foster mothers who were receiving AFDC because of shortages of foster homes and several other factors. The permanency planning movement and subsequent Child Welfare Reform Act of 1980 shifted policy toward placing children geographically closer and emphasized placement within the same cultural background. Foster parent recruitment efforts turned to inner city neighborhoods in order to meet the demand for homes for children of color (Garber et al., 1970; Kadushin, 1974). Kinship foster care was also greatly expanded as a result of the U.S. Supreme Court ruling in 1979 that enabled relative homes to receive the same reimbursement as non-relative homes (Boots and Geen, 1999).

"Welfare" became a racialized term at the historic conjuncture when women of color were able to claim the right to domestic motherhood through receipt of AFDC. Beginning in the 1970s, regressive political currents obtained growing influence, stimulating increased political support for welfare cutbacks and an assault on the political acceptability of entitlement. The passage of the Personal Responsibility and Work Opportunity Reconciliation Act of 1996 (PRWORA) was the culmination of the years of critique of the welfare system, and abolished the program, Aid to Families with Dependent Children (AFDC), the major source of support for poor women and children for the past 60 years.

The Challenges of Fostering

The foster care system cannot function without a pool of available foster mothers. Shortages of foster mothers have been documented for several decades (Child Welfare League, 1979; Campbell and Downs, 1987; Chamberlain et al., 1992; Pasztor and Wynne, 1995; Department of Health and Human Services, 2002). The reasons for the shortfall include the poor image of foster care, inferior pay, increases in working women and the inadequate support services for increasingly demanding care

(U.S. GAO, 1995; Boyle, 2002; Department of Health and Human Services, 2002).

Nevertheless, many foster mothers meet the challenge of caring for children who are among the most vulnerable children in our country (National Center for Children in Poverty, 2002). Studies have repeatedly shown that many of these children suffer from psychological, health, and educational deficits or delays (Zima et al., 2000; Chernoff et al., 1994; Pilowsky, 1995; Simms et al., 1999; Horwitz et al., 1994; Klee et al., 1997; Kortencamp and Ehrle, 2001; National Center for Children in Poverty, 2002). Foster mothers provide 24-hour care to children, are constantly on call to the child welfare agency in order to accept new placements, and are expected to be responsible for accompanying children to court dates, family visits, school appointments and medical, psychiatric and developmental services. Addressing the multitude of needs of foster children can be very demanding and time-consuming and foster children often require more assistance with activities of daily living than other children. Foster parents play a critical role in their foster children's lives, creating more impact than anyone else on the extent to which children in their care will be nurtured and protected.

Furthermore, insufficient attention has been paid to the fact that a high proportion of foster mothers are low-income women (Fein and Maluccio, 1991; Wozniak, 2002; Barth, 2001; Kortencamp and Ehrle, 2001; Orme and Buehler, 2001). Foster mothers are not paid for providing care, but receive monthly boarding rates to cover the costs of the children's upkeep calculated at the equivalent of a low-income level of support (USDA, 2000), reflecting the notion that caregiving should come from the heart, embracing self-sacrifice and eschewing monetary reward.

Motivation to Serve as a Foster Mother

Because caring for foster children is a difficult undertaking, it is valuable to ascertain what motivates women to become foster mothers. Reviews of major studies of foster mother motivation have identified two types of foster mothers, those who were more oriented to external motivation such as the desire to help someone else and other things related to social gratification and those motivated by internal or family-oriented reasons, such as gratification from their roles as mothers and companionship for oneself or one's children (Jones, 1985; Bell Associates, 1993). Other common motivations for becoming a foster mother include love of children, community service and a desire to supplement family income (Hampson and Tavormina, 1980; Seaberg and Harrigan, 1999). It has been noted that such motivations have changed little over time (Seaberg and Harrigan, 1999).

Combining welfare with foster mothering to supplement family income can also be understood as part of a survival strategy given the economic and family care realities of contemporary working class foster families (Swartz, 2004; Wozniak, 2002). Poor single mothers trying to balance paid work and caregiving face significant hardships and struggle to make ends meet (Edin and Lein, 1999; London, Scott, Edin and Hunter, 2001). Women turn to welfare when other support systems such as the labor market and the family have failed them and often "package" government assistance with other income sources in order to support their families (Edin and Lein, 1997). Fostering enables the option for such mothers to remain at home to care for children, yet contribute to the household economy by doing something rewarding and socially meaningful. Foster care board rates are low, yet the rates are much higher than the welfare grant and are fairly steady and predictable, so that it can enable such foster mothers to care for foster children and pay household expenses that assist the entire family (Wozniak, 2002).

METHODOLOGY

Study Goals

This study sought to explore the experiences and perceptions of foster mothers on TANF within the current climate of diminished support for caregiving in the context of welfare reform through several questions: How do foster mothers perceive the changes such as time limits and expectations that they enter the workforce in light of their responsibilities as foster mothers? Since fostering children is so challenging and undervalued, what rewards and successes of fostering do they identify? What do mothers identify as employment related goals upon leaving TANF and what options do they see available to them? Do they plan to continue serving as foster mothers?

Data Collection

The study was conducted as a telephone survey of 100 active foster mothers, both kinship and non-relative, serving with three private New York City foster care agencies. All of the foster mothers were currently caring for at least one foster child and had received Temporary Assistance for Needy Families within the past six months.

A convenience sample was utilized, drawn from lists of foster mothers provided by the foster care agencies who met the study criteria. A combination of procedures followed in order to enhance the response rate and ability to reach the population in question (Frey, 1983; Lavrakas, 1987) including the sending of an informative advance letter in English and Spanish to each person referred for participation and the concentration of interviews on early mornings, evenings and weekend hours when foster mothers were most available. Many initial refusals were successfully deterred by asking to set up a call-back appointment, since the refusal was often due to the inconvenience of the time of the call since foster mothers were often occupied with parenting responsibilities.

Contact was made or attempted with a total of 205 foster mothers drawn from the lists provided by the agencies in order to reach the desired sample of 100. Most non-responses were due to foster mothers' ineligibility to participate because they did not meet the study criteria. In fact, many of the foster mothers were pleased to be able to share their thoughts and many appeared genuinely sorry that they could not participate. Sixty-eight of the foster mothers contacted were not eligible to participate because they no longer fit the criteria. The complex dynamics of the welfare system, recent welfare reform policies and the child welfare system were fully evident. Reasons for ineligibility included that the foster mother was no longer on welfare, was now working, the foster home was inactive because children had been reunited with parents or adopted, or the foster mother had transferred to another type of assistance such as Supplemental Security Insurance (SSI) or Disability. It is noteworthy that there were only 9 refusals. Interviews lasted between 25 minutes and one and a half hours, with an average length of 40 minutes.

A structured survey was used that included a variety of Likert type, closed questions and well as a series of open-ended questions inquiring about foster mothers' perceptions of how the changes in welfare policies affected themselves, their foster parenting and the children in their care. The survey questionnaire was translated in order to accommodate foster parents whose primary language is Spanish. The process of double translation, a method considered the most adequate translation procedure, was utilized to produce the closest cultural equivalent of the instrument (Marin and Marin, 1991).

Data Analysis

The Statistical Package for the Social Sciences (SPSS) was used for the quantitative data analysis. Content analysis was performed on the qualitative data. The data was transcribed on note cards and analyzed by the method of constant comparison (Lincoln and Guba, 1985). The data was reviewed case by case in order to identify words, themes and concepts. Notes were made on the cards regarding the various themes and categories of responses that emerged. The cards were then sorted into similar themes to create categories. They were then reviewed and compared in order to isolate meaningful patterns and concepts, and analyzed in consideration of previous research and theories (Berg, 2004).

Limitations of the Study

Some study limitations stem from the fact that an availability sample was used and the research design did not include a comparison group or measurement at various time frames in order to measure change before and after the implementation of the new welfare regulations. The findings also relied on the self-report of the foster mothers and not actual observation of children's behavior or case records.

In spite of these limitations, this study uniquely examines foster mothering in the context of welfare reform. There are no other known studies about the topic. The study also makes a contribution to the body of knowledge about foster mothers. Most previous studies of foster mothers have examined issues of motivation, role perceptions and performance, satisfaction, challenges associated with fostering, recruitment and retention (Buehler, Cox and Cuddeback, 2003). Above all, this study enables the opportunity to hear directly from low-income foster mothers whose voices are rarely heard and less so are the voices of low-income, non-English speaking women.

RESULTS

Study Participants

The majority (64 percent) of the participants were Latina, with 32 percent African-American, 2 percent other and 1 percent White (see Table 1). Forty-nine respondents characterized their primary language as English, 31 as Spanish and 19 classified their households as other and specified

TABLE 1. Foster Mother Demographics

Characteristic	Frequency
Age of Foster Mother	
Mean Age	45.2
Median Age	46
Race and Ethnicity	
Percent Latina/Hispanic	64
Percent Black/African-American	32
Percent White	1
Percent Other	2
Language	
Primary Language	49
Percent English	31
Percent Spanish	19
Percent Bilingual English/Spanish	
Language of Survey	
Percent English	54
Percent Spanish	46
Length of Time as Foster Parent	
Mean Number of Years	5.12
Median Number of Years	3
Type of Placement	
Percent Non-Relative	60
Percent Kinship	38
Percent Both Non-Relative and Kinship	2
Educational Attainment	
Percent With 8th Grade or Less	29
Percent With 9th,10th or 11th Grade	36
Percent With High School Diploma or GED	17
Percent With Some College	11
Percent With Associates Degree	4
Percent With Bachelor's Degree	2
Welfare Receipt	21
Percent Receiving Welfare One Year of Less	19
Percent Receiving Welfare For Two Years	6
Percent Receiving Welfare For Three Years	14
Percent Receiving Welfare Five Years or More	61
Percent With Previous Time On Welfare	50

N = 99

bilingual in both English and Spanish. It appeared that a number of those in the bilingual category were not comfortable in English. Forty-six of the respondents opted to conduct the survey in Spanish, which is indicative of a more limited English proficiency among the respondents.

Educational attainment was low among the respondents in the study. A total of 65 percent of the foster mothers had not graduated from high school. Within this group, 29 percent of the foster mothers had completed eighth grade or less. In addition, Latinas and those foster mothers with limited English proficiency were most represented among those with lower levels of education.

Sixty percent of the respondents were non-relatives, 38 percent were relatives (kinship foster mothers) to their foster children; and 2 were caring for both relative and non-relative children. Sixty-one percent of the mothers had received welfare for five years or more and were facing time limits in the near future.

Heavy Caregiving Responsibilities

The family responsibilities of the foster mothers in this study exceed that of many other families (see Table 2). They were caring for total of 227 children. Thirty-three percent of the respondents were caring for only one foster child at the time of the interview, 32 percent were caring for two foster children, 19 percent were caring for three foster children, 14 percent were caring for four or five foster children, while two families cared for groups of six or seven children.

While these foster mothers are similar to other TANF families who have been found to have an average of two children (Department of Health and Human Services, 2000), their responsibilities extend additionally to their foster children who require higher levels of care than other children. The families in this study were caring for an average of two foster children in addition to an average of two of their own biological or adopted children, so that the average foster mother was caring for four children.

TABLE 2. Caregiving Responsibilities of Foster Mothers

Total Number of Foster Children	227
Mean Number of Foster Children	2.3
Number Ages 0-2 years	58
Number Ages 3-5 years	54
Number Ages 6-12 years	83
Number Ages 13-17 years	25
Number Ages 18-21 years	9
Total Number of Birth Children	188
Mean Number of Birth Children	2
Number Ages 5 years or less	17
Number Ages 6-12 years	77
Number Ages 13-21 years	94
Number Children Special/Exceptional Rate	36

One third of the respondents were caring for three to seven foster children in addition to their biological or adopted children. Consistent with the growing trend of younger children entering the foster care system (U.S. GAO, 1995, National Center for Children in Poverty, 2002), nearly half of the children being cared for by these foster parents were five or under.

More than one-third of the foster mothers were caring for at least one child who was classified as having special or exceptional needs. The types of problems and disabilities of their foster children included but were not limited to at least six children who were HIV positive, drug exposed children, severely acting out children with problems of fire-setting and Attention Deficit Hyperactive Disorder (ADHD), deafness, cerebral palsy, fetal alcohol syndrome and severe trauma such as abandonment and physical abuse.

Work Requirements and Foster Parenting

A series of questions explored foster mothers' attitudes toward work requirements and foster parenting (see Table 3). Two-thirds of the respondents did not believe it was fair to require foster mothers to work. Thirteen percent of the respondents found the question difficult to answer or were hesitant to express an opinion, perhaps reflective of the ambivalence about work and motherhood that is pervasive in our society. No one strongly agreed that it was fair to require foster mothers to work. Furthermore, a large proportion of the foster mothers expressed

TABLE 3. Foster Mothers' Attitudes Regarding Work Requirements and Foster Parenting

Attitudes Regarding Work Requirements	Frequency (Percent)
Fair to Require Foster Mothers To Work	
Strongly Disagree	30
Disagree	36
Agree	21
Strongly Agree	0
Don't Know	13
Foster Children Need a Foster Mother Providing Full-Time Care	
Strongly Disagree	2
Disagree	8
Agree	46
Strongly Agree	32
Don't Know	12
N = 100	

the belief that foster children need full-time care. One tenth disagreed and twelve percent did not know if foster children need a foster mother who is at home full-time caring for them.

Rewards and Successes of Fostering Children

Very high levels of rewards and satisfaction in fostering children were reported by the foster mothers, resulting in a mean score of forty-three on a scale with possible scores ranging from twelve to the forty-eight (see Table 4). The highest amount of gratification resulted from their role as mothers, such as helping children, companionship for oneself or one's children and the self-esteem and sense of accomplishment derived from their caring activities.

Extrinsic types of rewards were reported with less frequency. Reasons relating to external motivation or social gratification such as providing a community service and expression of religious values did not score as high as those other aspects of foster parenting rewards and successes. Obtaining training, learning things that could help obtain employment and supplementing the foster mother's income received the lowest ratings. Interestingly, the item that resulted in the lowest score was whether the foster board rates supplemented the foster parents' family income. Although nearly one-third of the foster mothers expressed

TABLE 4. Frequencies of Rewards and Successes for Foster Parents

	Not At All	A Little	Some	A Lot
Helping Children	0	2	2	95
Improves Feelings About Self	2	2	6	89
Use Mothering Skills/Talents	2	2	5	89
Provides Companionship	2	4	5	88
Sense of Accomplishment	2	1	9	85
Help Another Family	1	6	5	83
Learn Child Management	2	1	9	77
Provide Community Service	7	9	9	68
Get Training	5	14	21	58
Express Religious Values	14	14	11	58
Learn Things That Help Obtain Employment	14	15	15	46
Supplement Income	22	15	15	29

N = 99

rewards in this area, these results stand in sharp contrast to the very high amount of rewards and successes reported in the family-oriented types of rewards.

Further analysis was conducted in order to see if foster mothers' overall ratings of rewards and successes were associated with other variables such as ethnicity, primary language, type of placement, and number of children in the home (see Table 5). Although all foster mothers reported high levels of rewards and successes, some cultural differences emerged. Positive associations were found for ethnicity and language. Latina foster mothers and limited English speakers expressed higher levels of rewards and successes in their experiences foster mothers than African-American foster mothers. A positive association was also found to exist for foster mothers with more than four foster children placed in their homes than for those caring for fewer children, which was an unexpected finding. Counter intuitively, there was no association between the level of rewards and successes for foster mothers and the type of foster care placement.

Qualitative data from the open-ended questions offers richer insight into foster mothers' thoughts and perceptions about their roles as caregivers to foster children.

TABLE 5. Foster Mother Rewards and Successes by Ethnicity, Language, Type of Placement and Number of Foster Children

	Mean	SD	T	df	P
1. Ethnicity					
African American	41.7	2.7	2.49	74	.015*
Latina	43.9	3.7			
2. Language					
English	41.3	3.7	3.27	59	.002*
Spanish	44.25	3.1			
3. Type of Placement					
Kinship	42.6	4.3	.785	76	.435
Non-Relative	43.3	3.6			
4. Number of Foster Children		F			
One	42.4	2.831	78	.04*
Two	43.0				
Three	41.7				
Four or more	45.3				

Note: *p < .05
1, 2, 3 Significance levels pertain to result of T-test for equality of means
    4 Significance levels pertain to the result of one-way analysis of variance in which the post- hoc tests Tukey HSD confirmed a significant difference in rewards between foster mothers caring for four or more children

Children come first: A strong theme was the importance these mothers saw in caring for children and for many, a preference to remain at home to do it themselves, characterized by statements such as:

> I'm not sure if they are going to send me to work and I won't be available to take emergency placements of children. I would like to take care of more children.

> I liked working, but it was hard to be available for foster children. I prefer to stay at home and care for foster children.

Motherwork: Foster mothers frequently mothers referred to their fostering as work and saw it as an important service and responsibility that took much time and energy, yet was devalued and unrecognized. This foster mother who has dedicated the past for the past twelve years to fostering, adopted four special needs foster children and cares for another special needs foster child, as well as her own three children stated:

> Foster mothers make a sacrifice, especially those like me who do it as a career. I'm saving the city thousands of dollars by caring for kids with conduct disorders and other problems.

This kinship foster mother, caring for three children, two of whom are under five said:

> We foster parents have a 24 hour job, we should get paid for, it's very needed These children need love and attention and you can't give it to them if you are somewhere else.

Mothering Plus: Foster mothers continually made references to the exceptional needs of the children in their care and the amount of time and energy involved, illustrating how these responsibilities made participation in work outside the home very difficult.

A foster mother of a toddler with fetal alcohol syndrome explained:

> It's hard to try to do the two things at once, to work and be a foster parent. My foster child has many medical appointments and welfare is not sympathetic. It's a job being a foster parent and hard to juggle public assistance with being a foster parent.

As an African-American kinship foster mother of three children who are classified as special needs children indicated:

> It's hard to work and have children with many special needs. One foster child has ADHD (Attention Deficit Hyperactivity Disorder) and another had learning disabilities. It's hard to get to the schools when they get sick or have problems.

The following foster mother had been fostering for nearly 15 years. In her care were four foster children, as well as two adopted adolescents. Her fostering responsibilities included a mother-child placement, whereby a teen mother is placed with together with her baby with the goal of assisting the mother in assuming responsibility for her baby. These are considered to be among some of the most difficult placements to manage and therefore urgently needed by foster care agencies. She stated:

> I quit workfare and gave up my benefits because I had to be to work by 6:30 am and had to leave very early in the morning. It was hard to get the kids to school and the give my foster children the attention. I couldn't work and do that at the same time.

This foster mother who cares for four foster children, one under two as well as school-aged children who were classified as special needs due to ADHD explained:

> They don't understand that a foster parent needs to be home with the children, we have many responsibilities. There are a lot of appointments for therapy and the special needs of the children.

They also suggested that mandating foster mothers to work poses risks to foster children:

> I have a very difficult child with special needs. I almost have had to give him back but don't want to. You can't be on PA (public assistance) and try to work if you have disabled kids.

Making Ends Meet: As single mothers with limited opportunities in the labor market and lack of other supports, combining public assistance with fostering was a way to enable them to stay at home to care for their children as well as others needing care.

A foster mother who adopted one child from foster care and cares for a foster child below the age of two and her two school-aged birth children explained:

> I was working before, but I have young children and I thought that by being a foster mother I could stay home and care for others and also care for my own kids. I needed help–I have two kids and don't have family here to help, so I receive public assistance. I think it's better to stay home, someone is always there for them.

An older Spanish-speaking foster mother, 62 years of age with limited work experience and formal education, had been fostering for 13 years and managing by combining this with welfare assistance. She was caring for three foster children, one on medication for hyperactivity. Her fears are revealed about the end of welfare assistance:

> I'm worried about how I will pay the bills. I don't think I can work with the responsibility of the children. I think that being a foster mother to kids with so many needs is more work than going to work. I have to wait for three different buses for them every morning because they are all in special ed.

Another foster mother of eleven years with an education level below eighth grade, who cares for two relative foster children and two adopted children, stated:

> I'm not sure I'll be able to make it without welfare. I have health problems and need supports.

Positive aspects of work: While most foster mothers find the welfare work regulations difficult, some identified some helpful aspects of work which included personal satisfaction, improved self-esteem and respect and the belief that they were better parents by working and better role models for their children.

> Personally, it's helpful. It's my world, my time to myself. I'm not mom or grandma during this time. I think kids appreciate it when their mom is working. They appreciate the time we spend when I return, and I appreciate them too.

Several foster mothers felt that they were learning new skills and accumulating helpful vocational experience. One foster mother indicated: "I was getting experience, working with lawyers and learning valuable skills. I also got computer experience." Another foster mother's response demonstrates a positive attitude regarding work, yet reflects the lack of status accorded to caregiving: "I liked working and getting out, rather than being a homemaker. You can say do something and get more respect."

Future Employment

In consideration of the fact the foster mothers are expected to work upon reaching the five-year time limit, questions explored their employment interests. Foster mothers' employment interests reflected a heavy emphasis on caregiving work, especially caring for children, which was reported by 44 percent of the foster mothers. Another 14 percent stated that they wanted to care for the sick and elderly.

As might be expected, there was a great amount interest in work involving children. More than half were very interested in a job working with children and an additional 20 percent reported that they were interested in working with children when asked about specific interest in working with children.

Foster mothers expressed a strong commitment to remaining a foster parent, consistent with the high level of rewards and successes reported earlier (see Table 6). Projecting one and two years into the future, the majority of foster parents said that they were likely to continue to care for foster children. The majority of foster parents also stated that they would continue to care for foster children should they begin work, school or a training program or were no longer entitled to receive welfare benefits.

TABLE 6. Foster Parents' Plans to Continue Fostering

Continue To Care For Foster Children	Very Likely	Likely	Unlikely	Very Unlikely	Don't Know
One year from now N = 99	36	41	3	4	15
Two years from now N = 98	29	35	7	7	20
Begin Work, School, Training N = 97	33	36	4	7	17
No longer receive welfare N = 96	34	34	5	6	17

However, a significant proportion indicated that they did not know if they would continue, indicating that there is a possibility that they may decide not to foster in the future, especially if it becomes more difficult due to changed work/family circumstances.

DISCUSSION

Caregiving and Identity

The respondents in this study overwhelmingly attributed positive meaning to their experiences as foster mothers and wanted to be able to devote their time and energy to fostering children. They found validation of themselves in their roles and abilities as mothers and caregivers, which was reflected by more internal family-oriented reasons than those related to external motivation or social gratification. The greatest rewards and successes reported stemmed from feelings that they were helping children, using their skills as mothers and the self-esteem and sense of accomplishment derived from their caring activities. Several foster mothers pointed out that by fostering, they were able to do something they enjoyed that also had social value compared to other types of jobs that might be available to them given their educational and skill level, such as assignments in the Work Experience Program or working at McDonalds. Fostering was therefore consistent with their needs, interests and abilities and something they felt that they did well. Despite the culturally devalued social status of full-time mothers, and of foster mothers in general, these foster mothers found their caregiving to be a source of pride and sense of accomplishment. This is also a possible explanation for the higher level of gratification found among foster mothers caring for larger groups of children.

Some women's identity and conception of selfhood pivots around their ability and desire to give care and also contributes to their decision to receive welfare (Cancian and Oliker, 2000; Lewis, Carvalho and Nelson, 2001; Thornton-Dill et al., 2004). Such women view raising children as their primary commitment, identify as "nurturers" as opposed to "providers" and believe that working outside the home conflicts with parenting (Lewis, Carvalho and Nelson, 2001). In the wake of welfare reform, poor mothers no are longer able to determine for themselves how to balance their time between the dual responsibilities as caregivers and providers. Whatever limitations existed within previous policies, they enabled poor single women to make such choices for themselves (Mink, 1999, Sainsbury, 1996).

Welfare reform has accentuated the divides that exist among American women in terms of race and class. The fact that a majority middle class mothers work outside the home have been used as a justification for obligating poor single women to the same. Welfare reform policies are based on the notion that any job or even workfare is better than caring for dependent family members and renders the contributions of foster mothers invisible. Such policies not only removes vocational choice, but also deprives poor mothers of their right to choose how to manage their family's lives, creating yet another form of oppression.

Cultural Values and Gender Roles

Since a majority of the foster mothers were Latina and they found fostering to source of reward and success at the greatest levels, the influence of Latino cultural values and attitudes regarding gender roles and caregiving are considered in this discussion (Cruz, 1991; Quiroz and Tosca, 1992). While such values are never static and differ on the basis of factors such as level of education attainment and acculturation (Cooney and Ortiz, 1983; Kranau, Green and Valencia-Weber, 1982; Marin and Marin, 1991, it has been asserted that Latinas are less likely to participate in the labor-force than non-Latina white females due greater emphasis for women on family and having children than on personal accomplishments or work commitments (Cruz, 1991; Quiroz and Tosca, 1992; Rodriguez and Kirk, 2000). For these reasons, receipt of welfare should not be presumed to be a rejection of work, but a reflection of the value these mothers place on caring for their children themselves (Quiroz and Tosca, 1990; Cruz, 1991; DeParle, 1998; Starr, 1999). Evidence is also emerging that Latinas among those facing greatest obstacles transitioning from welfare (Rodriguez and Kirk, 2000). These include a lack of human capital and the added difficulty of acquiring the necessary human capital under current welfare reform regulations (Rodriguez and Kirk, 2000). Another stressor is the need for many women to recast gender roles and balance caretaking and providing for their families (Rodriguez and Kirk, 2000; Quiroz and Tosca, 1990; Cruz, 1991; Starr, 1999).

There is also a long tradition of a caregiving ethic in the African-American community, although such mothering has often taken place under conditions of oppression. Hill Collins (1991) asserts that among African-American women, motherhood, including the community "othermother" tradition of caring for unrelated children, is viewed as a symbol of power and recognition, often serving as a foundation for community building and activism.

Fostering: Undervalued and Underpaid

Foster mothers found fewer rewards in the foster care reimbursement and its ability to supplement family income. Numerous studies support the view that reimbursement rates for foster children are too low to adequately cover all of their expenses (Simon, 1975; DeJong and Specht, 1975; Kadushin, 1988; James Bell Associates, 1993; Department of Health and Human Services, 2002; Wozniak, 2002). Foster parents subsidize the foster care system through their volunteer time and out of pocket expenses (Pasztor, 1995; Meyer, 1988; Smith and Smith, 1990), placing greater burden on low-income foster mothers.

The lower rewards accorded to training and gaining employment skills also reflect the devalued status of foster mothers. Caregiving is devalued due to its relegation to the private sphere and because such work is often performed by women with low status with regard to race, class or immigration (Nakano Glenn, 2000; Folbre and Nelson, 2000). Foster mothers made frequent references to the work and difficulty involved in managing children with a complex variety of needs, yet fewer women regarded themselves as developing marketable skills. This is also reinforced by the systems in which they interact. Foster mothers are not considered foster care agency employees; the time they invest in training is not compensated and fostering does not lead to any type of professional recognition or career ladder. This invisibility was also apparent at the welfare office, where their experience had no bearing on employability assessments or the types of opportunities for work or training available to them.

The Future–Welfare to What?

An encouraging finding was the strong commitment and desire of these foster mothers to continue fostering children regardless of the welfare policy changes. However, they also clearly articulated the ways in which entering the labor market will make this effort increasingly difficult. Additional research found that entering paid employment has a negative impact on foster parent retention (Campbell and Downs, 1987; Rhodes, Orme, and Buehler, 2001). The notion that there are sufficient numbers of families with a parent at home willing and able to care for seriously troubled children entering the foster care system may be increasingly unrealistic as welfare reform unfolds.

Women's employment choices and how they choose to structure work and parenting in their lives are shaped by opportunities and constraints. The employment preferences of the foster mothers in this study are reflections of cultural and gender identity, but are also related to macro-level employment barriers such as occupational segregation (Cohen, 2004). As foster mothers confront the mandate of entering the labor market, there is strong evidence that they will engage in some type of caregiving work, such as child care, where they will earn exceptionally low wages and no benefits. The increased demand for child care services created by welfare reform work requirements has lead many foster parents to become childcare providers and has further decreased the numbers of available foster mothers (Malm et al., 2001). Child care is certainly needed for the increased numbers of working mothers, but encouraging this trend is shortsighted if the results are greater demands on foster mothers' time and less financial resources that ultimately shortchange foster children. Of equal alarm is the assumption that poor women are better off caring for other women's children rather than their own, particularly when such policies are carried out in the name of "family values." Under this scheme, foster mothers are doubly disadvantaged, because the care they provide to foster children and their birth children is treated as their "personal responsibility."

CONCLUSIONS

The desire to provide care to children is a central aspect of the identity of women such as these foster mothers and should be viewed as a positive attribute and social resource rather than a character defect that has been defined as "dependency" and in actuality involves the caring of others. Care of dependent persons, such as children, must be recognized as social contributions that require societal reciprocation (Kittay, 2001). The following are recommendations to address key issues regarding caregiving as TANF foster mothers confront welfare reform.

Improve Economic and Professional Status of Foster Mothers: The need for the reconstruction of foster care from a pretend natural family to an adequately compensated social service has been cited for nearly two decades (Meyer, 1985; Kamerman and Kahn, 1990). While there is no coordinated or government sponsored initiative to address this need, foster parents have been acknowledged as agency employees in some settings, with introduction of salaries and benefits (Testa and Rolock, 1999; Eheart and Power, 2000; Boyle, 2002). Successful models include paying foster parents recruited from the low-income neighborhoods in which the families with children in need of care reside; offering as well as child care, respite care and an array of services in addition to salaries; and training families receiving welfare assistance to serve as specialized foster parents to children with developmental disabilities (Casey Family Programs, 2001). Several states, partnering with community organizations, provide housing supports for low-income families that provide foster care through rental assistance and low-interest, no-down-payment mortgages (Boyle, 2002). Creating more non-poor foster parents through improved economic support makes sense (Barth, 2001). Recruitment is costly and time-consuming, many families are unwilling to care for the older and more troubled youth entering the system, resulting in continual shortage of appropriate homes and the lack of experienced caregivers.

Revision of Time Limits for Caregivers: The federal time limit structure within TANF can provide more flexibility in assisting working families by "stopping the clock" for those caring for young children, or going to school and increasing exemptions for those who cannot find and maintain employment due to barriers such as caring for a chronically ill or disabled child (Amey et al., 2000; Haskins et al., 2001; Phillips, 2002). "Earn-back" policies have been enacted in some states whereby work-related time limit exemptions given when a participant meets certain work thresholds. Under this policy, fostering could also be counted as employment at New York State's required number of hours of work participation and enable foster mothers to earn back benefit time (Phillips, 2002).

Ensure the Necessary Supports to Foster Mothers: Efforts should be made to ensure that TANF foster mothers continue to receive supports that they are eligible for, including food stamps, Medicaid, and child care and that they are not automatically dropped from these programs when they stop receiving cash assistance (Amey et al., 2000). Expansion of work supports that increase employment stability and to enable single mothers to sustain their employment and family obligations such as subsidized child care, paid family leave, and transportation assistance are sorely needed (Children's Defense Fund, 2000; Peterson, 2002). Child care has been found be one of the most pressing unmet service needs for foster parents (Zimmerman et al., 2000) and lack of daycare has a strong impact on foster mothers' decision-making about continuing as a foster parent (Rhodes, Orme, and Buehler, 2001). Foster mothers must compete with other low-income mothers and do not receive special consideration for child care services. Federal funding for child care services should be increased so that states can serve all children in low-income working families.

Policies must alleviate the burden on women such as these foster mothers by acknowledging the work involved in caring for high-risk children and how this impacts on their participation in the labor force. While such approaches may be more expensive, the social cost of inaction is tremendous, depriving foster children of the care they require and adversely affecting their caregivers (Buehler et al., 2003; Folbre and Nelson, 2000; Meyer, 2000; Women's Committee of 100, 2002). A change in the status of caregivers in our society is overdue and women, such as foster mothers, who care for children and dependent persons must be valued and supported in their efforts.

A policy that truly improves all women's opportunities as both workers and caregivers will ensure not only that all women have the rights and resources to be fairly rewarded in the labor market, but also offer the flexibility to decide how to balance market work and family needs. In the current political context of the United States, such policies seem out of reach, yet we must continually remind ourselves that most of these policies are commonplace in other industrialized countries and are critical for any advancement toward racial and gender equality and improved care for children.

REFERENCES

Abramovitz, M. (1988). *Regulating the lives of women*. Boston: South End Press.
Barth, R. (2001). Policy Implications of Family Characteristics. *Family Relations, 50*, 16-19.
Berg, B. (2004). Qualitative research methods for the social sciences. New York: Pearson Education, Inc.
Berrick et al. (1994). A comparison of kinship homes and foster family homes. *Children and Youth Services Review, 16*(1/2), 33-63.
Boots, S. and Geen, R. (1999). *Family care or foster care? How state policies affect kinship caregivers*. In the New Federalism: Series a, No. A-34, July 1999. Washington, D.C.: Urban Institute.
Boyle, P. (2002). "Is This Any Way to Treat Foster Parents?" *Youth Today, 11*(6), July/August 2002, 1.
Buehler, C. Cox, M.E. and Cuddeback, G. (2003). Foster parents' perceptions of factors that promote or inhibit successful fostering. *Qualitative Social Work, 2* (1): 61-83.
Campbell, C. and Downs, S. (1987). The impact of economic incentives on foster parents. *Social Service Review*. December, 599-610.

Casey Family Programs. (2001). *Resources on Professional Foster Parenting.* Washington, D.C.: Author.

Chamberlain, P. Moreland, S. and Reid, K. (1992). Enhanced services and stipends for foster parents: Effects on retention rates and outcomes for children. *Child Welfare, 71*(5), 387-401.

Cohen, P. (2004).The gender division of labor: "Keeping house" and occupational segregation in the United States. *Gender and Society, 18*(2), 239-252.

Cruz, J. (1991). *Implementing the family support act: The perspective of Puerto Rican clients.* Washington, D.C.: National Puerto Rican Coalition.

DeJong, G. and Specht, C. (1975). Setting foster care rates. *Public Welfare, 33,* 37-46.

De Parle, J. (1998). Welfare rolls show growing racial and urban imbalance. *New York Times,* July 27. p. 1.

Department of Health and Human Services, Office of the Inspector General. (2002). *Retaining Foster Parents.* Washington, D.C.: U.S. Government Printing Office, May.

Dubowitz, H., Feigelman, S. and Zuravin, S. (1993). A profile of kinship care. *Child Welfare, 72*(2), 153-169.

Dubowitz, H., Feigelman, S., Harrington, D., Starr, R. and Zuravin, S. (1994). Children in kinship care: How do they fare? *Children and Youth Services Review, 16,* 85-106.

Edin, K. and Lein, L. (1997). *Making Ends Meet: How single mothers survive welfare and low-wage work.* New York: Russell Sage Foundation.

Eheart, B. and Power, M. (2000). Hope for the children. In M. Harrington Meyer (Ed.) *Care work: Gender, labor and welfare states.* N.Y.: Routledge.

Fein, E. (1990). Issues in foster family care: Where do we stand? *American Journal of Orthopsychiatry, 61*(4), 578-583.

Fein, E., and Maluccio, A.N. (1991). Foster family care: Solution or problem? In W.A. Rhodes and W.K. Brown (Eds.) *Why some children succeed despite the odds.* New York: Praeger.

Fifield, A. and Halper, E. (1997). *Welfare's foster scare.* City Limits. May, 578-583.

Folbre, N. and Nelson, J. (2000). For love or money or both. *Journal of Economic Perspectives, 14*(4), 123-140.

Garber, M., Patrick, S. M., and Casal, L. (1970). The ghetto as a source of foster homes. *Child Welfare, 49,* 246-251.

George, V. and Wilding, P. (2002). Globalization and Human Welfare. London: Palgrave. Goerge, R. et al. (1995). *Foster care dynamics 1983-1993.* Chicago: Chapin Hall Center.

Gleeson, J. (1996). Kinship care as a child welfare service: The policy debate in an era of welfare reform. *Child Welfare.* Vol. LXXV, 41-49.

Gordon, L. (1990). The new feminist scholarship on the welfare state. In L. Gordon (ed.) *Women, The State and Welfare.* Madison: University of Wisconsin Press.

Halfon, N., Mendonca, A and Berkowitz, G. (1995). Health status of children in foster care: The experience of the Center for the Vulnerable Child. *Archives of Pediatric and Adolescent Medicine, 149,* 386-392.

Hampson. R. and Tavormina, J. (1980). Feedback from the experts: A study of foster mothers. *Social Work, 25*(2), 108-113.

Harrington Meyer, M. (2000). *Care work: Gender, labor and welfare states.* N.Y.: Routledge.

Hegar, R. and Scannapieco, M. (1995). From family duty to family policy: The evolution of kinship foster care. *Child Welfare*. Vol. LXXIV, 200-216.

Hill Collins, P. (1991). *Black Feminist Thought*. New York: Routledge.

Horwitz, S., Simms, M. and Farrington, R. (1994). Impact of developmental problems on young children's exits from foster care. *Journal of Developmental and Behavioral Pediatrics,15*, 105-110.

James Bell Associates. (1993). National Survey of Current and Former Foster Parents. Washington, D.C. Department of Health and Human Services, ACYF.

Kadushin, A. (1988). *Child welfare services*. New York: Macmillan.

Klee, L. (1997). Foster care's youngest: A preliminary report. *American Journal of Orthopsychiatry, 67*(2), 290-297.

Kortenkamp, K. and Ehrle, Jr. (2002). *The well-being of children involved with the child welfare system: A national overview*. Washington, D.C.: The Urban Institute.

Kraunau, E., Green. V., and Valencia-Weber (1982). *Hispanic Journal of the Behavioral Sciences, 4*(1), 21-40.

Lewis, D., Carvalho, I., and Nelson, B. (2001). *Identity, work and parenting: Implications for welfare reform*. Institute for Policy Research, Northwestern University.

Lincoln, Y and Guba, E. (1985). *Naturalistic inquiry*. California: Sage Publications.

Malm K., Bess R., Leos-Urbel, J. and Geen, R. (2001) *Running to keep in place: The continuing evolution of our nation's child welfare system*. Washington D.C.: Urban Institute.

Marin, G.and Marin, B. (1991). *Research with Hispanic populations*. Newbury Park: Sage Publications.

Meyer, C. (1985). A feminist perspective on family foster care: A redefinition of categories. *Child Welfare, 64*, 249-258.

Michel, S. (2000). Claiming the right to care. In M. Harrington Meyer (Ed.) *Care work: Gender, labor and welfare states*. N.Y.: Routledge.

Mink, G. (1998). Feminists, Welfare Reform, and Welfare Justice. *Social Justice, 25*(1), Spring, 1998.

Mink, G. (Ed.) (1999).Whose Welfare? Ithaca, N.Y.: Cornell University Press.

Nakano Glenn, E. (2000).Creating a caring society. *Contemporary Sociology,29*, 89-94.

National Center for Children in Poverty. (2002). *Improving the odds for the healthy development of young children in foster care*. NY: NCCP.

Oliker, S. (2000). Examining care at welfare's end. In M. Harrington Meyer (Ed.) *Care work: Gender, labor and welfare states*. NY: Routledge.

Orme, J. and Buehler, C. (2001). Foster Family Characteristics and Behavioral and Emotional Problems of Foster Children. *Family Relations, 50*, 16-19.

Pasztor, E. and Wynne, S. (1995). Foster retention and recruitment: State of the art in practice and policy. Washington, D.C.: CWLA.

Phillips, K. (2002). Earning Back Time: Who would benefit from work-related time limit exemptions? Washington, D.C.: Urban Institute.

Quiroz, J. and Tosca, R. (1992). For my children: Mexican-american women, work, and welfare. Washington, D.C.: National Council of La Raza.

Rhodes, K., Orme, J. and Buehler, C. (2001). A comparison of family foster parents who quit, consider quitting, and plan to quit fostering. *Social Service Review*, March, 84-114.

Rodriguez, E. and Kirk, H. (2000). National Council of La Raza. Issue Brief. Welfare Reform, TANF Caseload, and Latinos: A Preliminary Assessment. Washington D.C.: National Council of La Raza.

Sainsbury, D. (1996). Gender equality and welfare states. New York: University of Cambridge.

Scott, E., Edin, K., London, A and J. Mazelis. (2001). *My Children Come First: Welfare-Reliant Women's Post-TANF Views of Work-Family Trade-offs and Marriage.* Working Paper No. 4. New York: Manpower Demonstration Research Project.

Seaberg, J. and Harrigan, M. (1999). Foster families' functioning, experiences and views: Variations by race. *Children and Youth Services Review, 21,* 31-55.

Seccombe, K. (1999). *So you think I drive a cadillac? Welfare recipients' perspectives on the system and its reform.* Needham Heights, Mass.: Allyn and Bacon.

Sen, G. "Reproduction: The Feminist Challenge to Social Policy," in *Power and Decision: The Social Control of Reproduction.* Cambridge: Harvard School of Public Health 1994, 1-17.

Simms, M. D., Freundlich, M., Battistelli, E. S. and Kaufman, N. D. (1999). *Child Welfare.* Jan./Feb.166-183.

Simon, J. (1975). The effect of foster-care care payment levels on the number of foster children given homes. *Social Service Review.* Sept., 405-411.

Smith, B. and Smith, T. (1990). For love and money: Women as foster mothers. *Affilia, 5*(1), 66-80.

Starr, A. (1999). *Left behind: Everybody's leaving the welfare rolls–except Latinas.* The Washington Monthly, 31(4).

Swartz, T. (2004). Mothering for the state: Foster parenting and the challenges of government contracted carework. *Gender and Society, 18* (5), 567-587.

Testa, M. and Rolock, N. (1999). Professional foster care: A future worth pursuing? *Child Welfare.* Vol. LXXVIII (1), 108-124.

Thornton-Dill, B., Jones-DeWeever, and Schram, S. (2004). *Racial, ethnic and gender Disparities in Access to Jobs, Education and Training Under Welfare Reform.* University of Maryland: Consortium on Race Gender and Ethnicity.

U.S. General Accounting Office. (1995). *Child welfare: Complex needs strain capacity to provide services.* Washington, D.C. Author.

Zimmerman, E., Daykin,D., Moore, V., Wuu, C., and Li, J. (1998). Kinship and non-kinship foster care in New York City: Pathways and outcomes. N.Y.: United Way.

doi:10.1300/J137v15n04_04

The Effects of Residential Institutions on Adult Sexual Adjustment

William S. Rowe

SUMMARY. In many situations, for individuals that are institutionalized, normal sexual development is disrupted by among other things lack of privacy, gender separated living environment, lack of sex education, and lack of opportunity. Many institutions actively prohibit sexual expression and in other situations passively set the conditions for sexual assault and exploitation. These experiences in many cases have long-lasting and deleterious effects even after people return to the community. Recognizing that all people whatever their circumstances are sexual beings there is a need for explicit institutional policies that provide an atmosphere where sexual expression can be normalized as much as possible while ensuring a safe and supportive environment. doi:10.1300/J137v15n04_05 *[Article copies available for a fee from The Haworth Document Delivery Service: 1-800-HAWORTH. E-mail address: <docdelivery@haworthpress.com> Website: <http://www.HaworthPress.com> © 2007 by The Haworth Press, Inc. All rights reserved.]*

KEYWORDS. Institutions, sexuality, disability, sex education, sexual expression

---

William S. Rowe, DSW, is affiliated with School of Social Work, University of South Florida.

[Haworth co-indexing entry note]: "The Effects of Residential Institutions on Adult Sexual Adjustment." Rowe, William S. Co-published simultaneously in *Journal of Human Behavior in the Social Environment* (The Haworth Press, Inc.) Vol. 15, No. 4, 2007, pp. 81-92; and: *Adult Development and Well-Being: The Impact of Institutional Environments* (ed: Catherine N. Dulmus, and Karen M. Sowers) The Haworth Press, 2007, pp. 81-92. Single or multiple copies of this article are available for a fee from The Haworth Document Delivery Service [1-800-HAWORTH, 9:00 a.m. - 5:00 p.m. (EST). E-mail address: docdelivery@haworthpress. com].

INTRODUCTION

Institutions were originally established in order to protect their residents from harm and exploitation. The mentally ill, disabled, or orphaned were sent to asylums and orphanages in order to care for their needs and protect them from the dangers of indigent society. Institutions also served the purpose of protecting the community from the unsocialized, criminals, and diseases, such as tuberculosis, any of which could cause harm to the community at large. In medieval Europe, monasteries and convents provided this care. When England broke with the Roman church and dissolved the monasteries, the state was forced to take responsibility for hospitals and almshouses.

In the United States, most of these institutions were organized and administered by the state or religious orders, whether they be Catholics, Quakers, Lutherans, Salvation Army, etc. The first penitentiary in the United States was started by the Quakers. The term penitentiary actually derives from the word penitence. The Quakers believed that prison was a time to read the Bible and form a closer relationship with God. Other institutions, such as residential schools for Native American children and orphans, were run by religious orders to provide children with care, shelter, education, training and often assimilation.

Although these institutions were commonly established with the main goal of helping their residents, they eventually became corrupt, often physically and sexually abusing the very individuals they were meant to protect. The negative effects of the experiences in institutions on later sexual adjustment of adults have been devastating and far-reaching. They are seen in the therapist's office, the divorce court, psychiatric disorders, post-traumatic disorders and a series of other maladjustments including depression, suicide and sex offending.

Institutions were commonly gender separated into all male or all female facilities. Under these circumstances, there was little likelihood that normal sexual development and adjustment could occur for the residents (Johnson, 1975). In reviewing, what Johnson referred to as the three philosophies of institutions that care for the physically disabled he suggested that institutions were guided by either the eradicate, tolerate or celebrate philosophy of sexuality (Johnson, 1975). He suggested that most institutions adhered to the "eradicate" philosophy, which attempted to eradicate any possibility of sexual expression among the residents. This was ensured by there being no possibility of privacy in traditional group care and severe penalties or consequences for any residents engaging in sexual behavior. Johnson also suggested that the "tolerate" philosophy, which appeared to be more liberal (expressed as "we wouldn't disapprove as long as the sexual activity was socially appropriate") was really only the eradicate philosophy in disguise. Clearly, if severely physically disabled residents did not have the independent capacity to engage in sexual interaction, the tolerate philosophy would have the same result as the eradicate philosophy. Residents would not be able to engage in sexual behavior without support or assistance, and without access to privacy all sexual behavior would appear inappropriate. In essence both the eradicate and tolerate philosophies push sexual behavior underground, where it is more likely to become abusive and exploitive and result in immediate and long-term negative effects for the residents, even after they have left the institution.

He described a somewhat utopian situation where physically disabled residents who had few other pleasures available to them should be offered the opportunity to engage in mutually desirable sexual activity, which meant providing privacy, and in some cases, facilitating access for the residents who could not physically do this themselves. Clearly, Johnson was challenging normative thought and to this day only a few total care institutions mostly in Europe have embraced some of his ideas. This work will be limited to reviewing some of the key issues that occur in total care institutions in the United States that have serious effects on the sexual adjustment of adults who have resided in such facilities.

THE PRISON SYSTEM AND SEXUALITY

The first example of how institutions can negatively affect the sexual development of residents can be seen in our prison system. The prison sexuality policies call for the eradication of all sexual activity among inmates. This eradication of sexual behavior forces sexual activity underground. Sexuality in prisons is often distorted into a means of oppressing other inmates, and loses its natural purpose of fulfilling physical needs or helping to form intimate bonds. Sexual exploitation and rape are used as ways to assert power and control in the prison population. This negative use of sexuality can have devastating effects on the sexual development of an inmate. Once released from prison these experiences often lead them to engage in sexually deviant behaviors.

The subject of sex in prison is something that has been ignored by social scientists and society as well (Hensley, Struckman-Johnson, & Eigenberg, 2000). Sex in prison is performed both as an aggressive form of power gratification and as consensual sex for gratification

(Hensley et al., 2000 & Knowles, 1999). Many young boys and men are pressured into homosexuality by relentless sexual predators who use trickery, debt, and threats of physical harm (Fishman, 1934). Davis interviewed more than 3,000 inmates in the Philadelphia jail system, and he concluded that 3% of men were sexually assaulted in a 26 month period (Davis, 1982). The low percentage may reflect men's unwillingness to admit or even recognize accounts of sexual assault. Knowles believes that these aggressive sexual assaults may be fueled by racism or the desire to pick on the weaker or more feminine inmates (Knowles, 1999).

Consensual sex for gratification has also been researched, and studies have found the rate of consensual same-sex activity in prisons to be between 2 and 65 percent (Hensley, Tewksbury, & Wright, 2001). Again the wide variance may be attributed to the man's reticence to admit to homosexual acts. Studies have also found that 99% of inmates had masturbated, 38% had touched another male in a sexual way, 36% received oral sex from another inmate, and 32% performed anal sex on another male (Hensley et al., 2001). Overall the rate of consensual homosexual behavior increased after the inmates were incarcerated. Seventy nine percent of inmates claimed to be heterosexual, but that number decreased to 69% after release from prison (Hensley et al., 2001).

Religion has a strong influence on an inmate's likelihood of having consensual sex with another inmate. Non-protestants were more likely to engage in "sinful" behavior than protestant inmates (Hensley et al., 2001). This is due to the fact that the more conservative protestant church is more openly opposed to homosexuality. This negative attitude towards sexuality can also be seen in the Catholic Church when Pope John Paul II reaffirmed the church's position that masturbation is a sin that carries serious moral consequences (Rowe & Savage, 1987). Another influence on an inmate's likelihood of having consensual same-sex activity is the inmate's race. White inmates are more likely to engage in same-sex activity than non-whites (Hensley et al., 2001). The use of consensual sex activity in exchange for nonsexual goods and services can also affect the rates of sexual activity among inmates (Ward & Kassebaum, 1965).

These studies have shown that both aggressive and consensual sex activity are a part of prison life, regardless of any prison policy that calls for its eradication. Institutions should allow inmates to engage in autoerotic and consensual sex behavior without fear of punishment (Hensley et al., 2001). Masturbation provides a release for pent up tension and stress, and allowing consensual sex may reduce the amount of sexual oppression in prisons. Allowing married inmates a normal outlet for sexual release through conjugal visits would also help release tension and stress. A study by Giallombardo (1966) of a women's federal reformatory demonstrated that female inmates developed close emotional and familial links with each other (Giallombardo, 1966). They tended to satisfy each other's psychological, social, and physiological needs. Male inmates might be able to develop the kind of relationship that these female inmates have demonstrated if they were given the appropriate sexual outlets.

The experiences that inmates have while in prison clearly affect them when they are reintroduced into their community. Inmates who used sex as a form of oppression may continue to have abusive sexual relationships once they leave prison. Men who were forced to hide their consensual sex activity while in prison are socialized to think, through the institution, that sex is wrong or dirty. These men would most likely have trouble developing normal sexual relationships once they are out of prison. With the sole exception of specific programs for sexual offenders, probation, aftercare and halfway house programs almost exclusively avoid dealing the with sexual adjustment concerns of the ex-inmates.

NURSING HOMES/EXTENDED CARE FACILITIES

Other institutions that can negatively affect the sexuality of its residents are nursing homes or extendicare facilities. Middle adulthood, commonly referred to as "middle age," brings new physiological, psychological, and social changes. The female menopause, and the male climacteric often referred to as male menopause are often accompanied by diminished sexual interest. Most sexual problems occurring during middle age are rooted in these changes and can even be made worse by stereotypes of waning sexuality as a result of aging (Rowe & Savage, 1987). Recently, modern medications and aggressive advertising have begun to change this picture for people in their fifties and sixties but the sexuality of the elderly remains shrouded in the myth that sexual interest and desire decrease and literally disappear with age. These societal attitudes are the elderly's greatest barrier to sexual expression. Many elderly persons no longer have opportunities for private contact, because they live in segregated nursing homes or have been widowed and are without a partner (Rowe & Savage, 1987).

Intimate relationships are important to life satisfaction and physical health. Sexual expression can play an important role in the preservation of an older person's well-being, even when they are in a nursing home (Bauer and Geront, 1999). Residents of nursing homes have suffered many losses such as their homes, their health, and their independence. An intimate relationship is something a resident can still sustain and treasure (Atlanta Legal Aid Society, 2004). The elderly individuals' need for touching, pleasure, and intimacy do not change, but there are few socially acceptable means for them to realize these needs (Rowe & Savage, 1987). Expressions of sexual affection are often frowned upon by the adult children of the older persons and considered unseemly or lewd. Often they become the subject of ridicule by the staff and there are countless stories of elderly males exploiting the fact that they are greatly outnumbered by female residents.

DEVELOPMENTAL DISABILITIES

The situation is probably most insidious with persons with developmental disabilities. Many high functioning developmentally disabled individuals are able to translate their sexual expression into relationships during their adult years, but their sexuality is often unacknowledged and unexpressed (Rowe & Savage, 1987). Negative attitudes towards the sexuality of the developmentally disabled can be seen as early as 1614, when a physician named Montalto claimed that mental retardation could be caused by an over indulgence in sexual pleasure (Rowe & Savage, 1987). These negative attitudes continued throughout the 1930's and 1940's. Many institutions sterilized or castrated their residents to eliminate custodial problems with caring for menstruation and masturbation in female and male patients respectively. Some states even created sterilization laws for the developmentally disabled in an effort to support the eugenics movement and rid society of potentially more developmentally disabled people. These institutions became so proficient in this effort that in the 1930s, German physicians were sent to the study the techniques which were subsequently used in Nazi concentration camp. Negative reactions to the sexuality of the developmentally disabled can even be seen as late as the 1960's, when marriage was still illegal for retarded persons in 18 states.

Prohibitions against sexual expression for the developmentally disabled of all ages reinforce negative attitudes towards sexuality during later years. These negative attitudes make any sexual expression become viewed as distasteful and undignified. Commonly children with development disabilities first became institutionalized in their early adolescence when they began to express their sexual urges. This was frightening for the parents who were concerned about the possibility of pregnancy for the girls and potential legal implications for the boys whose unsocialized sexual advances were often misconstrued as aggression. Once the children were institutionalized, they commonly had strict prohibitions again any expressions of sexuality and received little or no sex education.

Subsequent to deinstitutionalization in the seventies and eighties, many of these former residents expressed a myriad of sexual adjustment problems. In other instances since many thought they would never live outside the institution again inappropriate expressions of sexuality (for example public masturbation) were left uncorrected. An example of one of the more disturbing stories came from my own practice when a high functioning developmentally disabled man expressed concern about his desire to expose himself in a local park. After many hours of treatment and investigation, it was later discovered and verified that as an adolescent in a total care institution for the developmentally disabled he was regularly sexually exploited by both the adult residents and the staff for years. None of which had ever been reported or debriefed. Clearly, his post institution adjustment has left him forever marred.

Case studies abound, with individuals who, subsequent to their sexually exploitive and abusive experiences in institutions, upon their return to the community went on to endure extraordinarily difficult circumstances. Many had no other means to support themselves other than prostitution but they did not have the sophistication or street smarts to protect themselves from pimps and pushers. As a result they were easily exploited often becoming drug addicted and infected with STDs and HIV.

Loneliness and pain can be amplified for patients in institutions, and it is quite natural for these patients to seek out intimacy and comfort (Deegan, 2001). We must find ways for this to occur in legitimate and non exploitive ways. A growing concern with human rights has led to a reexamination of the quality of life for special populations that have traditionally been cared for in institutions (Rowe & Savage, 1987). The developmentally disabled is one of the special populations whose rights are being reconsidered given the current focus on deinstitutionalization. The right to appropriate and satisfying sexual expression for this group has presented a perplexing challenge to individuals, families, and health care professionals. Many workers find they lack the adequate information and resources to respond to the sexual concerns of their developmentally disabled clients.

PHYSICAL AND MENTAL DISABILITIES

Many people have increasingly expressed concern that persons with disabilities are sexually disenfranchised, because society incorrectly perceives them as asexual (Milligan and Neufeldt, 2001). The myth that persons with disabilities are asexual is rooted in two primary lines of thinking. One line of thinking is that persons with disabilities have or are presumed to have a sexual dysfunction, and their gratification opportunities are considered limited. This idea leads many to believe that the sexual needs of people with disabilities are nonexistent or subjugated (Milligan and Neufeldt, 2001). Another line of thinking is that, although they may be sexually intact, their psychiatric disorders lead some to believe that they have limited social judgment and are unable to have responsible sexual relationships.

A study by McEvoy et al. (1983) has shown that sexual activity is in fact an important part of life for people with disabilities. This study of women diagnosed with schizophrenia in a long-term institution found that 65% of women reported having intercourse while in the hospital during the past three months (McEvoy, Hatcher, Applebaum, & Abenethy, 1983). A study by Warner et al. also demonstrated the presence of sexual activity in hospital mental health units. Warner et al. (1997) found that 30 of the 100 patients who participated in their survey (response rate 60%) reported engaging in some form of sexual activity (Warner, Pitts, Crawford, Serfaty, Prabhakaran, & Amin, 1997). Ten of these 30 participants reported having consensual sex. These studies clearly demonstrate that the disabled are not asexual beings, but should instead be seen as having normal desires for sexual activity. The psychosocial history of many institutionalized psychiatric patients reveals numerous instances of early sexual abuse and conflict regarding sexual orientation or normal developmental milestones. These circumstances provide a rationale for prohibiting sexual expression when what is needed in many cases is sex education, guidance, and support.

A similar situation exists for individuals in ill health. Most caregivers are comfortable providing empathy and support to people with terminal diseases but do not include an assessment of their sexual concerns as part of their role. Most hospice facilities and palliative care units focus on pain control, and family and spiritual concerns. Very few concern themselves with the intimacy needs or sexual expressions of their residents. This issue came into greater awareness early in the AIDS pandemic when relatively young people, who in some cases largely defined themselves by their sexuality, rapidly populated these units. These relatively young gay men wanted to be intimate with each other but this was difficult for the staff to accept. In the simplest of terms, a hospital room provides little privacy and a hospital bed seldom accommodates two people.

Society continues to deny or ignore the sexuality of people with disabilities. These discriminatory attitudes have negatively affected the ability of people with disabilities to begin and sustain sexual relationships (Milligan and Neufeldt, 2001). We have made significant gains in our biological and psychosocial understanding of sexuality in the context of disability, but we still have not done enough to effect change in the lives of people with disabilities. An increasingly vocal constituency of people with disabilities has become frustrated with the social barriers to their full participation in life, particularly in the area of sexuality.

PROMOTING SEXUAL HEALTH FOR CLIENTS

North American cultural norms influence us into thinking that sex is bad or immoral and sexual feelings or expressions of sexuality are wrong. These attitudes might be held by the assigned caretakers of people in institutions, and they may intervene into the sexual activities of their clients based on their own attitudes of what healthy sexuality should be (Rowe & Savage, 1987). A worker's attitude is an important influence in situational and organizational responses to the sexual behavior of clients. Negative attitudes of caregivers would lead to the neglect or suppression of the patient's sexual needs. This problem is made worse by the fact that many professional caregivers feel responsible for their clients instead of feeling responsible to their clients. This gives the professional a pseudo-parental stance that leads many of them to adopt a controlling rather than facilitative orientation.

The pressure to control clients' behavior tends to be accentuated in the area of client sexuality (Rowe and Savage, 1987). There is a strong tendency for staff members to assume responsibility for their clients' sexuality out of fear of pregnancy, sexual abuse, or sexual activity within a group home becoming public knowledge. This tendency to assume the responsibility of a client's sexuality usually takes precedence over opportunities to encourage clients to be responsible for their own sexual behavior.

The staff's controlling orientation does not allow the clients to communicate their sexual needs and wants, which is critical to a smooth passage through their sexual adjustment period. This can be even more frustrating for clients because interaction with potential sexual partners increases during this adjustment period that is described as a time of maximum sexual self-consciousness (Offer & Simon, 1976). A major task for these clients is to develop intimacy and solidarity rather than living in isolation, but the lack of sexual expression leaves many no options but to live in isolation.

The problem is not that patients want to engage in intimate relationships, but that institutions are stripping away their control over what they keep private and what they choose to make public (Deegan, 2001). Many hospitals have an obligatory policy statement regarding patient sexuality, but a policy prohibiting sex does not necessarily eliminate it. Buckley and Robben (2000) analyzed the sex policies of 31 state psychiatric hospitals in 16 states and found that 14 of these policies explicitly forbade inpatient sexual interaction, 12 stressed patient autonomy, and only 5 specified that staff should receive special training (Buckley & Robben, 2000). This research indicates that hospitals can have varied ways of approaching and managing their inpatients' sexual behavior. If one were to change this approach through the creation and implementation of new sex policies, one would allow the patients to retain their sexual freedom and dignity. The policy would be a guide that outlines the range of acceptable behavior for a particular group (Rowe & Savage, 1987). A sexuality policy would address the needs and right of the patient to search for intimacy, love, and physical comfort (Deegan, 2001). This policy must also address the institution's responsibility to protect the patient from the abusive and predatory behaviors of staff or other inpatients. This policy ought to consist of a sound knowledge base, an awareness of personal attitudes and a catalog of specific skills, and of which are fundamental components of competent professional practice in the area of human sexuality and the developmentally handicapped (Rowe & Savage, 1987).

A sexuality policy is helpful to both staff and clients alike. The policy gives the staff direction and supports them in their role as the provider of service (Rowe & Savage, 1987). It is also helpful to the client, because it brings consistency to day to day dealings. With a policy the client's sexual behavior is regulated by established rules, and not the particular attitudes about sexuality of the staff on duty.

In order to develop a sexuality policy, institutions must first identify the need for such a policy. The institution must then establish a committee to address the issue. Members of the committee should be selected from the various groups that will be affected by the policy (Rowe & Savage, 1987). It is crucial to include members of the Board of Directors in this committee since they are the group ultimately responsible for the philosophy, mandate, policies, and procedures of the agency. Representatives from the community agencies and advocacy groups that use or support the services of the agency should also be included in the committee. The sexuality policy must address areas such as: sex education, privacy, consent, sexual expression, sexual intercourse, masturbation, birth control, and sterilization.

Another important part of policy making is its implementation. There are several steps involved in translating policy into action. The first step is the formation of an advisory group (Rowe & Savage, 1987). In most agencies the second step is to hold a series of staff training sessions that will equip workers with the knowledge and skills necessary to implement the policy. Clients must be fully informed about the policy, the specific areas addressed in the policy, and its translation into rules governing behavior such as masturbation, sexual intercourse, the use of erotic materials, etc. In addition the policy should be made available to volunteers and other community agencies. A contact person should be identified who is available to answer and discuss questions regarding the policy. When the above tasks have been accomplished and the policy has been implemented, the advisory group is responsible for conducting periodic reviews. The review process involves soliciting feedback from advisory committee liaisons as well as from individuals. In any given review the feedback may lead to amendments to the original policy.

The development and implementation of policy is a complex, arduous and at times frustrating process (Rowe & Savage, 1987). Sexuality is an area fraught with myths and value-laden misinformation that generally evokes strong feelings. It therefore requires a creative and dedicated group of people to approach the task of developing and implementing a sexuality policy. With a proper sexuality policy, inpatients will be able to experience normal sexual development that will greatly help them as they mature and move on to their next stage in life. Under such circumstances, institutions could become solutions instead of the problems that have historically been the case.

REFERENCES

Atlanta Legal Aid Society (2004). Sexuality in the nursing home. Retrieved May 13, 2005, from http://www.atlantalegalaid.org/fact20.htm.

Bauer, M. & Geront, M. (1999). The use of humor in addressing the sexuality of elderly nursing home residents. *Sexuality and Disability, 17*(2).

Buckley, B.F. & Robben, T. (2000). A content analysis of state hospital policies in sex between inpatients. *Psychiatric Services, 51*(2), 243-245.

Davis, A.J. (1982). Sexual assaults in the Philadelphia prison system and sherriff's vans. In A.M. Scacco, Jr. (Ed.), *Male rape: A casebook of sexual aggressions* (pp. 107-120). New York: AMS Press.

Deegan, P.E. Human sexuality and mental illness: Consumer viewpoints and recovery principles. (2001). Retrieved on May 13, 2005, from Institutional Care website: http://www.intentionalcare.org/articles/articles_sex.pdf#search='effect%20%of%20institutions%20sexuality'

Fishman, J.F. (1934). Sex in prison: Revealing sex conditions in American prisons. New York: National Library.

Giallombardo, R. (1966). Society of women: A study of a woman's prison. New York: John Wiley.

Hensley, C., Struckman-Johnson, C., & Eigenberg, H.M. (2000). Introduction: The History of Prison Sex Research. *The Prison Journal, 80*(4), 360-367.

Hensley, C., Tewksbury, R., & Wright, J. (2001). Exploring the dynamics of masturbation and consensual same-sex activity within a male maximum security prison. *Journal of Men's Studies, 10*(1), 59.

Johnson, W.R. (1975). *Sex Education and Counseling of Special Groups.* Springfield, IL: Charles C. Thomas.

Knowles, G.J. (1999). Male prison rape: A search for causation and prevention. *The Howard Journal, 38*(3), 267-282.

McEvoy, J.P., Hatcher, A., Applebaum, P.S., & Abernethy, V. (1983). Chronic schizophrenic women's attitudes toward sex, pregnancy, birth control, and childrearing. *Hospital and Community Psychiatry, 34*(6), 536-539.

Milligan, M.S. & Neufeldt, A.H. (2001). The myth of asexuality: A survey of social and empirical evidence. *Sexuality and Disability, 19*(2).

Offer, D. & Simon, W. (1976). Sexual development. In Sadock, B., Kaplan, H., and Freedman, A. (eds.). *The sexual experience*, pp. 128-155. Baltimore: The Williams & Wilkins Co.

Rowe, W. & Savage, S. (1987). Sexuality and the developmentally handicapped: A guidebook for the health care professionals. The Edwin Mellen Press: Lewiston, New York and Queenston, Ontario.

Ward, D. & Kassebaum, G. (1965). Women's prison: Sex and social structure. Chicago: Aldine.

Warner, J., Pitts, N., Crawford, M.J., Serfaty, M., Prabhakaran, P., & Amin, R. (1997). Sexual activity among patients in psychiatric hospital wards. *Journal of the Royal Society of Medicine, 97*(10), 477-479.

doi:10.1300/J137v15n04_05

Examining the Perceptions of Grandparents Who Parent in Formal and Informal Kinship Care

Shelia G. Bunch
Brenda J. Eastman
Linner W. Griffin

SUMMARY. Child welfare workers are increasingly seeking formal kinship placements with grandparents when the child's biological parents can no longer provide a stable environment. Using a non-probability purposive sample (N = 55), this study explores whether or not caregiver well being is effected by the type of kinship care arrangement (formal vs. informal). The findings suggest that grandparents in formal kinship care arrangements experienced feelings of depression less often, were more satisfied with their parenting experiences and were observed to have a greater sense of satisfaction with life. Implications of these findings are discussed. doi:10.1300/J137v15n04_06 *[Article copies available for a fee from The Haworth Document Delivery Service: 1-800-HAWORTH. E-mail address: <docdelivery@haworthpress.com> Website: <http://www.HaworthPress. com> © 2007 by The Haworth Press, Inc. All rights reserved.]*

KEYWORDS. Child welfare, kinship care, elderly caregivers

Shelia G. Bunch, PhD, Brenda J. Eastman, PhD, and Linner W. Griffin, EdD, are affiliated with East Carolina University, School of Social Work, Greenville, NC.

[Haworth co-indexing entry note]: "Examining the Perceptions of Grandparents Who Parent in Formal and Informal Kinship Care." Bunch, Shelia G., Brenda J. Eastman, and Linner W. Griffin. Co-published simultaneously in *Journal of Human Behavior in the Social Environment* (The Haworth Press, Inc.) Vol. 15, No. 4, 2007, pp. 93-105; and: *Adult Development and Well-Being: The Impact of Institutional Environments* (ed: Catherine N. Dulmus, and Karen M. Sowers) The Haworth Press, 2007, pp. 93-105. Single or multiple copies of this article are available for a fee from The Haworth Document Delivery Service [1-800-HAWORTH, 9:00 a.m. - 5:00 p.m. (EST). E-mail address: docdelivery@haworthpress.com].

Available online at http://jhbse.haworthpress.com
doi:10.1300/J137v15n04_06

INTRODUCTION

Child welfare systems traditionally seek placements for children among kinship networks when the child's biological parents can no longer provide a stable environment. As a result of this practice, grandparents are increasingly, assuming full-time parenting responsibilities for their grandchildren. According to U.S. Census data, 2.4 million children were living with grandparent caregivers and 39% of grandparent caregivers had cared for their grandchildren for 5 or more years (U.S. Census Bureau, 2003).

Intergenerational caregiving historically has been a common occurrence among African American families, however, this social phenomenon is increasing for all racial and ethnic groups (Brown & Boyce-Mathis 2000; Whitley, Kelly & Sipe, 2001).

Grandparents intervene to circumvent temporary or permanent placement of their grandchildren into the child welfare system (Minkler & Roe 1993, Sands & Goldberg-Glen, 1998). Several studies have documented the mitigating factors that lead grandparents to assume primary care for their grandchildren. A major factor has been the proliferation of the drug epidemic in this country (Dowdell, 1995; Kelly, 1993; Minkler and Roe, 1993). Sands and Goldberg-Glen (1998) found that 71% of their sample of 123 caregiving grandmothers assumed care because their children were incapacitated by drug use. Dowdell (1995) found 80% of the grandmothers in their study were caregiving because of the drug use of their children. The incarceration of parents (Dowdell, 1995; Dressel & Barnhill, 1994), parental abuse and neglect (Minkler & Roe, 1993) and the illness and death of an HIV infected parent (Linsk & Mason, 2004) have also influenced the emergence of this new and evolving family structure.

As a result of assuming these responsibilities, grandparents experience a great deal of stress that could impact the quality of their own lives as well as their ability to provide quality care to their grandchildren. Grandparents raising grandchildren also present challenges to child welfare workers as they consider the feasibility of placing children with grandparents with physical and mental health risks (Sands & Goldberg-Glen, 1998). The health and psychological well-being of grandparents are important factors to consider when child welfare workers are seeking placements for children. The ability of the grandparents to assume and sustain the caregiving is essential to providing a stable environment that is conducive to the physical and emotional well-being of children. Children in these situations have been traumatized and may feel a sense of safety and stability with their grandparents that was not present when they were living with their parents (Daly & Glenwick, 2000). Given these factors, child welfare institutions should develop strategies for helping custodial grandparents cope with the lifestyle negotiations of integrating the needs of their grandchildren into their daily routines.

CHALLENGES AND DILEMMAS

Grandparents who assume parental responsibility for a "second time around" experience a new set of challenges and dilemmas. The challenge of assuming full-time responsibility for grandchildren impacts the lifestyles and daily routines of grandparents, (Dowdell, 1995; Sands & Goldberg-Glen, 1998). The traditional expectations of grandparenthood are often shattered with the assumption of full-time parenting for another generation of children. They may have anticipated a life free of full-time childcare to explore new avenues and adventures (Daly & Glenwick, 2000; Orb & Davey, 2005) such as spending more time with their spouses, continuing their education or having fun (Haglund, 2000).

Many of the factors related to rearing one's grandchildren include physical and psychological stress and the lack of economic resources and social support (Kelly, Beatrice, Whitley & Sipes, 2001) especially if they are caring for grandchildren with emotional, neurological, and physical problems (Daly & Glenwick, 2000; Dowdell, 1995; Szinovacz, DeViney & Atkinson, 1999). Some grandparents report that they have less time for themselves and that the quality of their friendships and marriages are compromised (Standridge & Floyd, 2000).

Some grandparents use caregiving the second time around to rectify past parenting mistakes (Roe, Minkler & Barnwell, 1994) while others feel anger or resentment toward their adult child for failing to care for their own children. The mental health of grandparents as parents may be impacted by the previous life experiences of grandparents when they were raising their own children (Kelly et al., 2001).

The stressors related to caregiver burden disproportionately affect women since they overwhelmingly assume care for their grandchildren (Dowdell, 1995; Sands & Goldberg-Glen, 1998). These grandparents are most likely to be single, aging women with limited resources. Fuller-Thomson and Minkler (2000) found that three-fourths of their caregiving grandmothers were not living with a partner and more than half lived below the poverty line. According to the U.S. Census Bureau

(2003), 19% of grandparent caregivers had incomes below the poverty level in 1999 with southern states reporting that 21% of grandparent caregivers were living in poverty.

HEALTH

The physical demands of raising a child in later life pose some special health concerns that negatively impact the physical and emotional well-being of grandparents (Landry, 1999; Musil, 1998). Many studies report that grandparents raising grandchildren experience diminished physical and emotional functioning, however, the research findings on the impact of caregiving on grandparents' physical and mental health are inconsistent.

Several empirical investigations have documented the relationship between caregiving and health. The grandparent may have difficulty meeting the physical demands of parenting. Whitley, Kelly and Sipe (2001) in their sample of 100 African American grandmothers found that 45% rated their health as fair or poor and many were at risk for serious health problems because of negative health behaviors related to diet and exercise. Sands and Goldberg-Glen (1998) found that 65% of their study sample was managing chronic health conditions such as high blood pressure and 25% identified a decline in physical health after assuming parental responsibilities for their grandchild.

Other studies found that custodial grandparents were impacted by health problems that contributed to functional limitations in their activities of daily living. However, the studies were not able to discern if the limitations were exacerbated by their caregiving role or were more salient because of the caregiving. (Fuller-Thomson & Minkler, 2000: Minkler & Fuller-Thomson, 1999). Perceptions of physical health may impact how one feels about other aspects of their lives. Dowdell's (1995) findings of serious health problems in caregiving grandmothers are consistent with other studies, however, the grandmothers in this study also reported poor self esteem, perceived their health as worse and did not feel supported.

The consequences of caregiving can compromise the treatment of illness and chronic disease of custodial grandparents because they do not interrupt their caregiving responsibilities to seek health care for themselves. The demands of caregiving can interfere with the ability to keep their own health care appointments and thereby jeopardize their own health by ignoring important symptoms or failing to seek care. Research by Minkler and Fuller-Thomson (1999) document the determination and perseverance of grandparents to continue their caregiving efforts in spite of the presence of physical symptoms or chronic conditions.

MENTAL HEALTH

There is a growing body of empirical evidence to support the idea that surrogate grandparenting has a negative impact on psychological well-being (Szinovacz et al., 1999). Minkler and Roe (1993) found that 37 percent of grandmothers raising grandchildren reported that their psychological health had deteriorated since assuming full-time caregiving. Kelly, Whitley, Sipe and Yorker (2000) found that 30% of their sample reported psychological distress scores in the clinical range resulting from limited resources, lack of support and poor physical health.

Mental health issues faced by grandparents in general tend to stem from the lifestyle negotiations they make to incorporate full time caregiving into their daily routine. Psychological stress and anxiety are exacerbated by several factors that impact the lifestyle negotiations of custodial grandparents (Musil, 1998). Many grandparents have little time to sustain relationships with social and community networks and they often report a loss of freedom and social isolation (Minkler, Fuller-Thomson, Miller & Driver, 1997). Some may feel that they do not receive adequate support from spouses or other family members. Minkler and Roe (1993) found that urban African American custodial grandmothers did not perceive their husbands or partners to be a source of consistent help with child rearing. Other grandparents are coping with the events that culminated with assuming care of their grandchildren (Minkler et al., 1997) as well as struggling with conflictual relationships with their own children (Sands & Goldberg-Glen, 2000). Grandparents may also experience stress when they are negotiating services with schools and other social service agencies. Financial circumstances are exacerbated by limited income and the difficulties associated with maintaining full-time employment (Sands & Goldberg-Glen, 1998).

Age may emerge as a significant variable when researchers examine the relationships between surrogate grandparenting and psychological distress. The age of the grandparent and the age of the child when grandparents assumed care can contribute to psychological distress, especially if older grandparents are caring for very young children (Whitley et al., 2001). Older adults might find caregiving stressful because they are vulnerable to the onset of health problems such as hypertension and diabetes or they may be coping with the loss of a spouse (Sands & Goldberg-Glen, 2000). Younger grandparents are also vulnerable to stress and psychological anxiety because they are more likely to work and manage multiple roles as well as caregiving responsibilities (Goldberg-Glen & Sands, 2000; Minkler et al., 1997).

The behavioral characteristics of grandchildren may also contribute to the psychological stress experienced by grandparent caregivers. Brown and Boyce-Mathis (2000) found that grandparents caring for children with physical or mental health problems or special educational needs were more likely to report lower scores on indicators measuring mental well-being than those whose child had no problems.

In a comparison of clinic and non-clinic grandparents seeking psychological services for their grandchildren, Daly and Glenwick (2000) found that clinic grandmothers reported more depression, parenting stress and poor parenting satisfaction than non-clinic grandmothers.

Depression is one of the more enduring effects of caregiving and elevated rates of depression among grandparent caregivers is a consistent research finding (Brown & Boyce-Mathis, 2000; Minkler & Roe, 1993; Musil, 1998). Fuller-Thomson and Minkler (2000) report that the depression may be triggered by the sorrow of coping with the distressing circumstances surrounding the onset of care such as substance abuse, incarceration, or death of their adult child. Minkler and associates (1997) found that caregiving grandmothers were almost twice as likely to be categorized as depressed as non-care giving grandparents, even after controlling for depression before the placement. Roe, Minkler, Saunders, and Fuller-Thomson (1996) reported inconsistent results given that some of their respondents reported depressive symptoms while others reported an improvement in their psychological well-being since assuming caregiving.

To date, a substantial portion of the research conducted on caregiving by older adults has focused on stress, depression, and other negative outcomes and studies on factors associated with the positive well-being of older caregivers is not well developed (Sands, Goldber-Glen, & Thornton, 2005). The MacArthur Study of Successful Aging found that the possession of external resources is just as important to enabling older caregivers to successfully manage their lives so as to experience well-being and life satisfaction as the possession of internal resources (Sands et al., 2005). Given this omission, this study seeks to explore whether or not caregiver well-being is affected by the type of kinship care arrangement (i.e., formal versus informal kinship care) that an older caregiver assumes child care responsibility.

METHODS

Participants

A non-probability purposive sampling technique was utilized to recruit participants for the survey. Investigators identified organizations in rural localities hosting support groups for grandparents raising their grandchildren in rural localities of Maryland, North Carolina, and Virginia and then contacted the administrative personnel in each organization. For this study, the term rural is defined in a general manner as being characterized by a low population density and not containing a metropolitan statistical area with a population greater than 250,000. Once contacted, the purpose of the study as well as procedures was explained and agency cooperation in recruiting potential participants was solicited. Written information was then forwarded to cooperating agencies so that potential participants could be told about the study. An investigator would then visit the agency, once again provide information about the goals of the study, the role of the survey interview, and request participation. Upon the indication of consent, a direct contact protocol was implemented. Both the participant and researcher had copies of the instruments. The researcher read the questions aloud while the participant marked their answers on the reply sheet provided. Recruitment of participants took place over a six month interval and yielded a sample size of 55. Participants were identified as belonging to one of 2 groups: the first group consisted of providers of formal kinship care (n = 23) where the child's placement in the relative's home was arranged by social services and resources were provided for the care of the child; while the remaining group were providers of informal kinship care (n = 32) where arrangements for care were made between family members and no resources were provided by social services.

Measures

The instrument used in this study was a multi-faceted questionnaire, comprised of a brief questionnaire developed by the investigators and three self report instruments assessing participant satisfaction with life, parental satisfaction, and depression. The study questionnaire gathered demographic information from the participants such as age, race, marital status, education level, employment status, and health status. Background information gathered included information about the circumstances necessitating the assumption of child care, number of children being cared for, length of time as a caregiver, contact with child's parent, custody status, whether or not formal assistance is received from social services for providing care, caregiver perceptions about available social resources, and the perceived impact providing care has had on their interpersonal relationships. Three social researchers reviewed the questions developed by the investigators to insure content validity.

The Satisfaction with Life Scale (Diener, Emmons, Larsen, & Griffin, 1994) is comprised of five items assessing the cognitive-judgemental aspects of general life satisfaction. Unlike measures that apply some external standard, the Satisfaction with Life Scale (SWLS) reveals the individual's own judgment of his or her quality of life. Respondents read each statement and respond using a 7 point Likert Scale ranging from "strongly disagree" to "strongly agree." Item scores are summed for a total score, which ranges from 5 to 35, with higher scores reflecting more satisfaction with life. The authors report that the SWLS's internal consistency is very good, with an alpha of .87 and good test-retest reliability with a correlation of .82 for a two month period. Concurrent validity was tested with varying adult samples reflecting young and older adult populations, while the authors reported that scores correlated with nine measures of subjective well-being, no further data was provided.

Depression was assessed using the Geriatric Depression Scale Short Form (Sheikh & Yesavage, 1986), a 15-item self-rating scale developed specifically for screening depression in the elderly. Respondents answer each of the items with a yes or no in relation to how they have felt over the past few weeks. Scores can range from 0 to 15 with a cutoff point of equal to or greater than 7 suggesting a large number of depressive symptoms. The reliability and validity of the instrument are good, with an internal consistency reliability of .89, a test-retest reliability of .85, criterion-related validity of .95 and concurrent validity of .96.

The Kansas Parental Satisfaction Scale (KPS) is a 3 item instrument designed to measure satisfaction with oneself as a parent, the behavior of one's children, and a person's relationship with the child. Items are rated using a 7 point Likert scale, responses are summed and can range from 3 to 21 with higher scores indicating satisfaction with one's parenting. The KPS has very good internal consistency, with alphas that range from .78 to .85. The author (Schumm & Hall, 1994) reports that KPS has good concurrent validity, correlating significantly with marital satisfaction and the Rosenberg Self-Esteem Scale.

RESULTS

Table 1 summarizes the demographic and background information for participants in the study as a whole. The majority of participants were African American (65%), not married (63.6%), and reported their status as either being a homemaker or retired. Overall, educational attainment for the sample was low, with the majority of the sample noting their educational attainment as either being high school or less. Approximately one third of the participants (33%) reported that they were either married or living with a partner. The majority of grandparents who participated in this study became caregivers more frequently as a result of issues of abuse or neglect (24%) or marital discourse (20%). Other issues resulting in the assumption of parenting included health related issues of the parent, substance abuse of the parent, parent incarceration, military deployment, or death.

Data analysis was conducted in two stages. An initial analysis was conducted to assess comparability of the two groups using demographic and background variables with no significant differences observed between groups as a result of this process. Once comparability of the two groups was addressed, t-tests for independent samples were performed on each measure. A summary of the results for each measure are presented in Table 2. Significant differences were observed between the two groups on all three measures. Caregivers in formal kinship care arrangements as a whole were observed to have fewer indications that they were experiencing feelings of depression, appeared to be more satisfied with their parenting, and were observed as having a greater sense of satisfaction with life. For the sample as a whole, GDS participant scores ranged from 2 to 14, with a mean score of 7.87 and a standard deviation of 4.57. Scores on the KPS ranged from 4 to 21 with a mean of 11.07 with a standard deviation of 5.79. Scores on the SWLS ranged from 5 to 24 with a mean score of 13.18 and a standard deviation of 6.28.

CONCLUSIONS/IMPLICATIONS

While the child welfare system must assess the physical and mental capability of grandparents to assume care of their grandchildren, agencies should also ensure that kinship placements with grandparents include program strategies that increase positive outcomes for both caregiver and child. As the number of aging grandparents who assume parenting responsibilities increases, it is important that we attempt to understand

TABLE 1. Demographic and Background Characteristics of Careproviders (N=55)

Item	n	%
Age grouping		
40 to 49	5	9.1
50 to 59	24	43.6
60 to 69	23	41.8
70+	3	5.5
Marital Status		
Never married	15	27.3
Married	20	36.4
Divorced	8	14.5
Separated	3	5.5
Widowed	9	16.3
Race		
Caucasian	17	30.9
African American	35	63.6
Latino	3	5.5
Education		
Less than High School	21	38.2
High School	24	43.6
Some College	10	18.2
Employment		
Working full-time	8	14.5
Working part-time	11	20.0
Homemaker	22	40.0
Retired	10	18.2
Unemployed	4	7.3
Self Report on Health Status		
Good	12	21.8
Fair	34	61.8
Poor	9	16.4
Reason for assuming caregiving role		
Abuse/Neglect	13	23.6
Health	7	12.7
Substance Abuse	9	16.4
Marital issues of parent	11	20.0
Incarceration	5	9.0
Deployment (military)	5	9.0
Death of parent	3	5.5
Relocation	2	3.6
Number of Children being cared for		
One	34	61.8
Two	16	29.1
Three	3	5.5
Four	2	3.6
Length of time providing care		
1 year or less	10	18.2
1 to 3 years	20	36.4
3 to 5 years	16	29.1
More than 5 years	9	16.4
Caregiver has regular contact with child's parent		
Yes	35	63.6
No	19	34.5

TABLE 2. Group Differences for Geriatric Depression Scale (GDS), Kansas Parental Satisfaction Scale (KPS), and Satisfaction with Life Scale (SWLS)

Measure	Formal Kinship Care n = 23		Informal Kinship Care n = 32		
	M	SD	M	SD	t (53)
GDS	6.66	4.08	8.17	5.27	−.410*
KPS	14.34	5.06	11.05	4.04	.976*
SWLS	13.72	6.20	10.43	6.46	.745*

*$p < .01$

caregiving grandparents from a positive perspective. In this study, we attempted to compared the perceptions of two groups of caregiving grandparents about their careproviding experience. Grandparents in formal kinship care arrangements appeared to have more positive outcomes on variables associated with well-being than grandparents who entered into informal kinship care arrangements.

The focus of this study was placed on assessing the possible influence the child welfare system could have from a non-deficit perspective. However, its findings need to be interpreted cautiously and several limitations should be noted. Participant responses to the study's questionnaire are subject to personal biases and distortions characteristic of self administered surveys. Secondly, participants are from one rural region in the Southeast, therefore responses need to be interpreted within that context and not thought indicative of all rural localities. In addition, the survey instrument was constructed by the authors for the study; therefore issues of reliability and validity remain. Thus, conclusive statements about the total kinship care provider population cannot be made. Future research efforts could be helpful in delineating what mediating factors play the largest role in caregiver outcomes.

The information gathered in this study has implications for working with multigenerational families in applied settings. The outcomes for grandparents providing care for their grandchildren were significantly impacted by the presence of external resources. The literature on caregiving grandparents well-being have generally focused on the negative impact that caregiving has on sense of satisfaction, satisfaction with parenting relationship, physical health, and mental health with particular attention given to depressive symptomotogy (Sands et al., 2005).

By emphasizing a perspective based on strengths, social workers should conceptualize caring for one's grandchildren as a choice and that can contribute to successful aging and child cargiving. The findings suggest that social workers in the child welfare system can best help grandparents caregivers by employing strategies that embrace a holistic perspective. By promoting connections for both the grandparent as well as the child, agencies would be congruent with the signficant body of literature that links well-being and resilience in both positive aging and child development.

REFERENCES

Brown, D. R. and Boyce-Mathis, A. (2000). Surrogate Parenting Across Generations: African American women caring for a child with special needs. *Journal of Mental Health and Aging, 6*(4), 339-351.

Daly, S. L. and Glenwick, D. S. (2000). Personal adjustment of grandchild behavior in custodial grandmothers. *Journal of Clinical Child Psychology, 29*(1), 108-118.

Diener, D., Emmons, R., Larsen, R., & Griffin, S. (1994). Satisfaction with Life Scale. In J. Fischer, & K. Corcoran (Eds.) *Measures for Clinical Practice: A Sourcebook. Vol. 2* (2nd ed., pp 501-502). New York, NY: The Free Press.

Dowdell, E. B. (1995). Caregiver Burden: Grandparents raising their high risk grandchildren. *Journal of Psychosocial Nursing, 33*(3), 27-30.

Dressel, P. L. & Barnhill, S. K. (1994). Reframing gerontological thought and practice: The case of grandmothers with daughters in prison. *The Gerontologist, 34*, 685-691.

Fuller-Thomson and Minkler. (2000). African American grandparents raising grandchildren: A national profile of demographic and health characteristics. *Health & Social Work, 25*(2), 109-118.

Haglund, K. (2000). Parenting a second time around: An ethnography of African American grandmothers parenting grandchildren due to parental cocaine abuse. *Journal of Family Nursing, 6*(2), 120-135.

Kelly, S. J. (1993). Caregiver stress in grandparents raising grandchildren. *IMAGE: Journal of Nursing Scholarship, 25*(4), 331-337.

Kelly, S. J., Whitley, D., Sipe, T. A., & Yorker, B. C. (2000). Psychological distress in grandmother kinship care providers: The role of resources, social support and physical health. *Child Abuse & Neglect, 24*(3), 311-321.

Landry, L. (1999). Research into action: Recommended intervention strategies for grandparent caregivers. *Family Relations, 48*(4), 381-390.

Linsk, N. & Mason, S. (2004). Stresses on grandparents and other relatives caring for children affected by HIV/AIDS. *Health and Social Work, 29*(2), 127-136.

Minkler, M. and Fuller-Thomson, E. (1999). The health of grandparents raising grandchildren: Results of a national study. *American Journal of Public Health, 89*(9), 1384-1388.

Minkler, M., Fuller-Thomson, E., Miller, D. & Driver, D. (1997). Depression in grandparents raising grandchildren. *Archives of Family Medicine, 6*, 445-452.

Musil, C. (1998). Health, stress, coping and social support in grandmother caregivers. *Health Care for Women International, 19*(5), p. 441, 15 pages.

Orb, A. & Davey, M. (2005). Research: Grandparents parenting their grandchildren. *Austrailian Journal on Ageing, 24*(3), 162-168.

Roe, K. M., Minkler, M., Saunders, F. & Thomson, G. E. (1996). Health of grandmothers raising children of the crack cocaine epidemic. *Medical Care, 34*(11), 1072-1084.

Sands, R. G. & Goldberg-Glen, R. S. (1998). The impact of employment and serious illness on grandmothers who are raising their grandchildren. *Journal of Women & Aging, 10*(3), 41-58.

Sands, R. G. & Goldberg-Glen, R. S. (2000). Factors associated with stress among grandparents raising their grandchildren. *Family Relations, 49*, 97-105.

Sands, R. G., Goldber-Glen, R. S., & Thornton, P. L. (2005). Factors associated with the positive well-being of grandparents caring for their grandchildren. *Journal of Gerontological Social Work, 45*, 65-81.

Schuum, W., & Hall, J. (1994). Kansas Parental Satisfaction Scale. In J. Fischer & K. Corcoran (Eds.) *Measures for Clinical Practice: A Sourcebook. Vol. 2* (2nd ed., pp. 501-502). New York, NY: The Free Press.

Sheikh, J., & Yesavage J. (1986). Geriatric Depression Scale (GDS): Recent evidence and development of a shorter version. *Clinical Gerontology: A Guide to Assessment and Intervention*, 165-173, NY: The Haworth Press.

Szinovacz, M. E., DeViney, S. & Atkinson, M. P. (1999). Effects of surrogate parenting on grandparents' well-being. *Journals of Gerontology, 54B*(6), S376-S388.

U.S. Census Bureau (2003). Grandparents living with grandchildren: 2000. www.census.gov/prod/2003pubs/ck-31.pdf. Retrieved 11-14-05.

Whitley, D. M., Kelley, S. J. & Sipe, T. A. (2001). Grandmothers raising grandchildren: Are they at increased risk of health problems? *Health and Social Work, 26*(2), 105-114.

doi:10.1300/J137v15n04_06

The Impact of Hopelessness and Hope on the Social Work Profession

Andrea K. McCarter

SUMMARY. Burnout and turnover are detrimental to social service organizations, social service providers and clients. Very often organizational characteristics are part of the cause for burnout. Burnout in a job can lead to hopelessness for social service providers and begin a vicious cycle of continued burnout and increased hopelessness. Knowing the characteristics of hopelessness can help social welfare institutions nurture their employee's level of hope thus impacting the way the social service providers work with their clients. doi:10.1300/J137v15n04_07 *[Article copies available for a fee from The Haworth Document Delivery Service: 1-800-HAWORTH. E-mail address: <docdelivery@haworthpress.com> Website: <http://www.HaworthPress.com> © 2007 by The Haworth Press, Inc. All rights reserved.]*

KEYWORDS. Hope, hopelessness, burnout

WORKPLACE EFFECTS ON SERVICE PROVIDERS: A LOOK AT HOPELESSNESS AND HOPE

The prevalence and incidence of burnout in social work is unknown, but considered to be an "above average risk of burnout" (Jayaratne &

Andrea K. McCarter, CMSW, is affiliated with The University of Tennessee, College of Social Work, 219 Henson Hall, Knoxville, TN 37916 (E-mail: akmccarter@comcast.net).

[Haworth co-indexing entry note]: "The Impact of Hopelessness and Hope on the Social Work Profession." McCarter, Andrea K. Co-published simultaneously in *Journal of Human Behavior in the Social Environment* (The Haworth Press, Inc.) Vol. 15, No. 4, 2007, pp. 107-124; and: *Adult Development and Well-Being: The Impact of Institutional Environments* (ed: Catherine N. Dulmus, and Karen M. Sowers) The Haworth Press, 2007, pp. 107-124. Single or multiple copies of this article are available for a fee from The Haworth Document Delivery Service [1-800-HAWORTH, 9:00 a.m. - 5:00 p.m. (EST). E-mail address: docdelivery@haworthpress.com].

Available online at http://jhbse.haworthpress.com
© 2007 by The Haworth Press, Inc. All rights reserved.
doi:10.1300/J137v15n04_07

Chess, 1984; Pines & Kafry, 1978; Soderfeldt, Soderfeldt, & Warg, 1995, p. 638). The financial, personal and social costs of burnout, although incalculable, are assumed to be of immense proportions and can be devastating to both the individual, the organization and the profession (Sowers-Hoag & Thyer, 1987). Burnout effects can cause depression and physical health problems in social workers.

These problems can potentially lead to social worker turnover or wastage. Knapp, Harissis and Missiakoulos (1981) discuss two terms in regards to turnover: turnover being defined as the loss of an individual in a specific social work job to another social work job and wastage being defined as the loss of an individual from the profession. The costs of turnover are high in separation (exit of an employee), replacement (interviewing and hiring) and training (time and money) for an organization as well as potential reinforcement of mistrust among the clients and decreased morale of the remaining employees (Blankertz, 1997; Braddock & Mitchell, 1992; Mor Barak, Nissly, & Levin, 2001).

Between 30% and 60% of social workers leave their jobs or change careers each year (Geurts, Shaufeli, & De Jonge, 1998; Jayaratne & Chess, 1984). Turnover in social work has "grave implications for quality, consistency and stability of services" (Mor Barak, Nissly, & Levin, 2001). Clients have reported that turnover or change of service providers causes personal disruption or prolonged crisis (Drake & Yadarma, 1996; Knapp, Harissis, & Missiakoulos, 1981). Additionally, turnover portrays a negative reputation of the profession. Burnout and turnover rates are extremely high in the social service fields partly because of feelings of hopelessness (Walsh, 1987).

A person's potential to become burned out can be influenced by her/his work environment, clients and their own characteristics (Soderfelt, Soderfelt, & Warg, 1995). Burnout was greatly researched in the 1980s and shown to have numerous causes. Outcomes of this body of research indicated that low work autonomy (Arches, 1991), lack of job challenge (Himle, Jayaratne, & Thyness (1986), low support (Jayaratne, Himle, & Chess, 1988), role ambiguity (Justice, Gold, & Klein, 1981), low salary and professional self-esteem (LeCroy & Rank, 1986), negative attitudes toward agency (Streepy, 1981; Fahs Beck, 1987) and difficulty in providing services (Fahs Beck, 1986; Streepy, 1981) are all work place reasons for burnout. These work place characteristics can result in a provider feeling a sense of fatigue or frustration (Freudenberger & Richelson, 1980), disengagement from the job (Cherniss, 1980), physical depletion (Pines, Aronson, & Kafry, 1981) and emotional exhaustion (Maslach & Jackson, 1981). There are number of suggestions that have been offered to prevent burnout such as improving staff communications, defining work roles and offering support (Fahs Beck, 1987; Hagen, 1989; Jayaratne et al., 1988) adequate training and mentorship (Corcoran & Bryce, 1983; Gibson, McGrath, & Reid, 1989) and increased financial resources (Gibson, McGrath, & Reid, 1989).

Burnout is of great concern because it is often contagious being passed from clients to staff, staff to staff, or staff to clients (Edlewich, 1980). Burnout from these work related characteristics can then lead to a risk of a provider feeling a sense of helplessness and hopelessness (Farran, Herth & Popovitch, 1995; Pines, Aronson, & Kafry, 1981).

Hopelessness has been shown to have detrimental effects on people ranging from increased physical health problems to depression and psychological problems (Grossarth-Maticek, Kanazir, Vetter, & Schmidt, 1983; Itzhaky & Lipschitz-Elhawi, 2004). Increased incidence of cancer, depression and suicidal thoughts are just a few of the problems people with a low level of hope may deal with. These impacts can lead to decreased functioning further lowering a person's level of hope. Many of the clients that social service providers work with are experiencing the physical and psychological effect of hopelessness. Social service providers who work with people who feel hopeless have the potential to taking on those traits of hopelessness. Likewise, a social service provider who is already experiencing a lack of hope can transfer that hopelessness to her/his clients.

Hopelessness can be considered as a way of feeling and acting (Farran, Herth, & Popovich, 1995). A person's hope can be threatened by being around others with low levels of hope, depleted energy, isolation, physical deterioration, concurrent losses and lack of information or feelings of devaluation (Farran, Herth, & Popovich, 1995). It is believed that hopelessness begins in childhood and develops throughout a person's life if there is not intervention (Erikson, 1982; Schmale, 1964). Hopelessness can leave a person feeling discouraged, despaired, deenergized, entrapped by situations with the inability to form concrete plan and realize different paths to reaching goals (Farran, Herth, & Popovich, 1995). Hopelessness causes impaired thinking and leads a person to have low expectations. There are a number of characteristics that can clue one into the fact that a person is experiencing hopelessness such as: social withdrawal, psychological discomfort, feelings of incompetence and being overwhelmed (Farran, Herth, & Popovich, 1995).

In the long run hopelessness has been shown to be detrimental in a number of ways. Hopelessness is a direct link to mental illness, depression and suicidal ideation (Beck, Kovacs, & Weissman, 1975; Fromm,

1968). People experiencing hopelessness also have an increased incidence of physical health problems, especially cancer (Frankl, 1963; Grossarth-Maticek, Kanazir, Vetter, & Schmidt, 1983; Richter, 1957). All of these detrimental impacts lead to a decreased ability to function thus creating unsuccessful attainment of goals. Specific to the social services field are issues of transference of hope from the social worker to the client or patient (Itzhaky & Lipschitz-Elhawi, 2004). There has been minimal literature related to hope and coping in social service literature and only in the medical social service field with AIDS patients. Even within this paucity of literature there is only one article discussing the level of hope among social service providers. Itzhaky and Lipschitz-Elhawi (2004) report that social service providers working with terminally ill patients often see things get worse with their clients and begin to have feelings of hopelessness and despair themselves which is then passed on to their clients.

The strengths perspective is one of the most popular approaches to social service practice and could be used in considering ways to break the cycle of hopelessness. It was developed as a response to the pathology model in which therapeutic focus was on the problem rather than possibilities. Barker (1999) defines strengths perspective as an "orientation that emphasizes the client's resources, capabilities, support systems, and motivations to meet challenges and overcome adversity" (p. 468). Although the strengths perspective has been defined in a variety of ways, there are five basic tenets of the model: (1) individuals have the capacity to grow, (2) focusing on strengths will enable individuals to grow, (3) individuals do the best they can, (4) human behavior is complex, making it difficult to predict behavior, and (5) clients know what is best for them (Staudt, Howard, & Drake, 2001; Weick, Rapp, Sullivan, & Kirsthard, 1989). The strengths perspective is just that rather than being extended into an intervention for clients or service providers.

Social workers need to feel hopeful on the job to provide good services to their clients. There are a number of reasons that this lack of hope is detrimental to social work, however the primary reason is that when social workers leave their jobs there is a disruption in the continuity of services to clients (Drake & Yadama, 1996). "Hope is a vital ingredient for enhancing quality of life and promoting health and healing" (Beck, Rawlins, & Williams,1984; Farran, Herth, & Popovich, 1995, p. 80; Farran & Popovich, 1990; Miller & Powers, 1988; Owen, 1989). The Code of Ethics presents guidelines indicating that the well-being of clients is the first and foremost important issue to social workers and the profession (NASW, 1999, 1.01). We cannot give to others what we don't have within ourselves (Elliott, 2005). If we want the best for our clients, then the well-being and best interest of the workers needs to be considered.

A step beyond strengths perspective would be assessing a person's strengths in an effort to guide her/him toward setting goals which is a primary part of hope theory. Hope theory is a more defined method that considers specifically evaluating a person's strengths, considering her/ his systems of support and ability to propel her/him toward a goal. Once a person's agency or motivation, pathways and goals have been determined a social service provider can evaluate and assess with the client how to increase or maintain the person's level of hope. In order to work with the strengths and hope of a client, the strengths and hope of the social service provider must be considered. Creating goals and evaluating agency and pathways can be developed as an intervention with clients and social service providers to increase a person's level of hope. Hope has promise in the social service field in identifying hopelessness in order to alleviate burnout and turnover. However, there needs to be appropriate measurement tools that are valid and reliable in social services.

Hope is the relationship between motivation and methods used in order to reach goals successfully. Hope provides the "stuff" that facilitates change in people. It provides the substance for making change and reaching goals. It is important for social service providers in that an ability to determine hope allows one to better assess a person's strengths and guide her/him through improvement. On an organizational level, there is a need for assessment of social service provider's level of hope in order to better determine ways to consistently maintain social service providers in the field, thus decreasing risks to clients.

In discussions of human development many suggestions have been created and tested to develop and increase hope as a person grows and matures (i.e., using positive self talk, learning to laugh at oneself, making and maintaining friendships, viewing problems as a challenge). There are a number of factors that play into a person's level of hope being high or raised: feelings of connectedness and a sense of control, having uplifting memories and affirmation of worth, have the ability to set goals and refocus time and have a number of cognitive strategies to reach goals (Farran, Herth, & Popovich, 1995). Additionally, a person's lightheartedness and other personal attributes play a role in her/his level of hope (Farran, Herth, & Popovich, 1995). According to Itzhaky and Lipschitz-Elhawi (2004) the role of a social service provider's supervisor and approach to supervision can have an impact on the provider's level of hope. Using analytical and cognitive approaches in providing education and support to the provider can help the person feel more hopeful in her/his job.

Hope Theory Definition Development

Historically, hope has not been clearly defined with terms that can be used in a variety of disciplines. Hope is primarily a way of thinking, but emotions do play a role in the level of hope that a person maintains (Elliot, 2005; Snyder, 2002). Hope is a positive expectation for reaching goals (Frankl, 1992; Stotland, 1969). One of the first theoretical definitions provided is that hope is "an expectation greater than zero of achieving a goal" (Stotland, 1969, p. 2). Nowotny (1989) reported a belief that "hope is activated when [people] encounter stressful events" (Snyder, 1998, p. 423) and that hope is made up of "inner readiness, active involvement, spiritual beliefs, relations to others perceived future possibilities, and confidence in desired outcomes (p. 423). Hope has also been defined hope as a construct "[involving] the realistic perception of upcoming positive outcomes, a feeling of confidence about one's plans to achieve goals, and the recognition of the importance of the interaction between self, others, and spiritual matters" (Herth, 1991; Snyder, 1998, p. 423). Hope is value neutral and is not the same as trust, virtues or values (Snyder, 2002).

"Hope is a positive motivational state that is based on an interactively derived sense of successful (a) agency (goal-directed energy), and (b) pathways (planning to meet goals)" (Snyder, Irving, & Anderson, 1991, p. 287). This definition was created for use in the psychology discipline and appears to be most fitting with social work. Hope is an interaction of a person's agency and pathways in relation to successful goal attainment (successful accomplishment)/obtainment (getting a desired object).

Goals can be discussed in terms of positive goals and negative goals. Positive goals are those things that can be achieved for the first time (i.e., graduation), maintenance of current situation (i.e., doing assignments and attending class) and increasing current situation (i.e., participation in study groups and extra credit activities). Negative goals are those things that one can achieve to deter from happening (i.e., being fired from a job) or to delay from happening (i.e., being laid off from work). Goals fall into three categories of functioning: repair, maintenance and enhancement. Repair goals are set in order to fill a gap (i.e., registering for a required course). Ongoing goals are those things that are day to day focuses (i.e., studying for a class). Enhancement goals include overall desires to be sought (i.e., graduation).

FIGURE 1. GAP Interaction

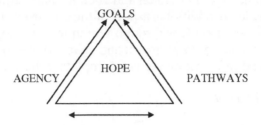

People set goals for things that they either want to attain or accomplish. Once those goals are set they determine pathways to direct their work toward those goals. The pathways and alternative pathways lead to a person's agency. A person's agency also plays a role in the development of pathways (see Figure 1). Successful attainment of goals will then lead to the initiation of other goals, thus creating a cycle. Agency has been described as the motivation or willpower that a person has to make her/his goals known. Agency indicates a capacity to use pathways and have alternative pathways to reach goals. In more layman terms agency is the energy and motivation that one has that her/his goals will be met.

Pathways or waypower are the methods and planning that a person will conduct in order to meet goals. The routes and alternative routes to attaining goal achievement are the way power or pathways. The can give a visual of thinking about how to get from point A to point B.

Hope is also defined as either being trait hope or state hope. Trait hope is that hope that someone has that is natural. It is lasting and enduring regardless of situations. It is related to how a person approaches life (Elliot, 2005; Farran, Herth, & Popovitch, 1995). The second type of hope, state hope, is more transient, and changes depending on the circumstances in which one is being asked to acknowledge her/his level of hope. State hope gives an indication of how hopeful a person feels about a current situation (Elliot, 2005; Farran, Herth, & Popovitch, 1995).

Hope began as a divine virtue before moving into the philosophical arena of discussion. Beyond being discussed hope was able to move into a more secular realm and become more of a scientific theme. Hope has since been considered an individual attribute that has been debated to be either stable or transient. Hope has been discussed as a vital outcome and mental state of individuals. Finally, hope has been most recently researched as a ubiquitous construct (Bloch, 1986) meaning that it is multifaceted: emotional and cognitive, involuntary and voluntary, subjective and objective, individual and social. Each definition and theory of hope provides an additional aspect of the construct. The different definitions provide a new lens through which to view hope. Hope definitions and explanations have grown and changed over time, but previous definitions and information are not completely discarded for the new.

Measurement Tools

In the past thirty years multiple tools have been created to measure the construct hope, however, the development of hope measurement instruments is still in the early stages (Farran, Herth, & Popovitch, 1995) and the tools are continuously being refined. All but one of the tools is self report survey instruments and range from 8-60 items. All of the items on the surveys are Likert type scale questions. These instruments vary in terms of complexity based on length and wording. Each of the tools has been created for research in the clinical populations (medical and psychological).

Stotland (1969) cited flaws with self report measures of hope being that the questions lend confusion for the responders. Also, as some of the instruments are long, it is difficult to ascertain the accuracy of the results when the scales are used with populations that are suffering physically or psychologically. Gottschalk (1974) attempted to alleviate these effects in using interviews and observations. It is the only verbal analysis scale and requires extensive training on the scoring component of using the scale in research (Farran, Herth, & Popovich, 1995). The Snyder scales (Snyder et al., 1991) were developed with consideration given to participants fatigue level and attention span. Snyder's hope scales account for these flaws in creating scales that have only twelve and eight items that are one line phrase items.

The scales that have been created over the past 30 years have been used primarily in the medical field. Most of the scales are more than 16 years old. The Herth Hope Scales (1991) have been used for the past 16 years, but there have been minimal studies conducted (Farran, Herth, & Popovich, 1995). The scales have not been used long term or with varied populations.

Research has been conducted for 15 years with various populations, using the Snyder Trait Hope Scale consistently. This research includes a number of populations including college students, psychiatric patients, veterans, cancer and spinal cord injuries patients and drug rehabilitation patients. Overall, the Snyder Hope Scales have been used consistently with multiple populations over the longest period of time.

Many of the scale developers have struggled with determining if hope is stable or transient. The Snyder scales account for each of these characteristics in that there is a scale for stable hope (State Hope Scale) as well as for dispositional hope (Trait Hope Scale) (Farran, Herth, & Popovich, 1995).

The majority of the measurement tools were developed for use in the medical field. Three of the scales were developed for use with college students and psychiatric patients. Although the alpha reliability scores of the measurement tools are above average, the Snyder scales have demonstrated increased levels of reliability consistently with different populations and as determined by varied researchers.

Snyder Hope Scales

The State Hope Scale, formally titled "Goals Scale for the Present," consists of six items that are answered on an eight point Likert scale. The scale is comprised of three agency questions and three pathways questions. Each question is worded in a positive tone and computes a score indicating the level of hope a person has at the moment of the testing. Higher scores equal higher levels of overall. The overall scale has been found to have a range of coefficient alphas to be = .82-.95 (Snyder et al., 1996). The scale is made up of two subscales in which a tester can determine a person's level of pathway thinking with a coefficient alphas = .74-.93 and agency thinking with coefficient alphas = .83-.95 (Snyder et al., 1996).

The Trait Hope Scale or "The Future Scale" was created to be used with adults and has been tested in a number of arenas ranging from college students to psychiatric patients and in the medical field to measure the stable level of hope a person holds. The original Trait Hope Scale was created with 45 items. The first research conducted with the scale was with psychology students at the University of Kansas (Harris, 1988). The original scale consisted of a 4 point Likert scale. After the preliminary analysis the scale was reduced to 14 items. The 4 agency items and 4 pathways items with the highest item remainder coefficients (>.20) were kept in the scale. There were 4 filler items added.

The current scale has twelve items to be answered on an eight point Likert scale. There are four questions related to pathways, four questions related to agency and four questions that are filler questions. Cronbach's alphas for the overall Hope Scale range from

.74-.88. The agency subscale has been shown to have a Cronbach's alpha range from .70-.84 and from .63-.86 on the Pathways subscale (Cramer & Dyrkacz, 1998; Snyder et al., 1991; Sumerlin, 1997).

Research Outcomes

Over the past three decades there has been an increased interest in hope and its impacts on people. This interest began in the medical field and has become a more interdisciplinary interest. Much of the research related to hope has been conducted in the medical profession beginning in the early part of the 20th century. Hope theory has been further defined and researched in psychology in the past twenty years.

Hope has been examined in a variety of populations including: cancer survivors and current cancer patients, people with terminal illnesses, burn victims, victims of racism, victims of violence, college students in both academics and athletics, outpatient mental health clients, combat veterans, elementary to high school students. There has also been research conducted to determine the differences of hope levels between men and women as well as the characteristic differences of high hope versus low hope people.

As a basic beginning to research on hope in the social service fields, Snyder (1989) began looking at stress, coping and the opposite of excusing. He worked with a number of researchers and offered a specific definition for hope in 1991 (Snyder, Irving & Anderson, 1991). There have been numerous scales created to measure hope in other disciplines primarily in the medical field. The Trait Hope Scale and State Hope Scales were developed to measure hope with psychiatric patients and college students aiding the transition of hope as a construct to hope as a theory. Hope has been discussed and researched in many areas including religion, mythology and philosophy, medicine, societal and political arenas, and academics. Arenas in which hope has been discussed has changed over time depending on what is societal importance at the time.

Qualitative research has been conducted looking at hope since the late 1960s. Initial quantitative, empirical research with hope has its roots in the medical field. Data has been collected through the use of interview, observations, group discussions and open ended questionnaires. Almost all of the qualitative research has been conducted in the medical field, with only 5 being in other areas. This medical research has been performed with adolescent and elderly oncology patients, children with disabilities and HIV patients. Other qualitative research has been conducted with college students and adolescent substance abuse. Additionally, there have been only two studies conducted primarily with people of a culture other than American. Averill, Catlin, and Chon (1990) did research comparing American and Korean college students). Qualitative research was also done with critically ill Korean patients (Chung, 1990). There have been no multi cultural quantitative studies published. All of the qualitative studies had less than 60 participants except the studies with non medical participants (N = 150) and those used open ended questionnaire methods. These studies considered a variety of variables: physical symptoms, anxiety, depression, social support, religion/spirituality, mental health, personal control, coping, treatment settings, self esteem, life satisfaction, social and medical history and caregiver characteristics.

Farran, Herth and Popovich (1995) compiled a review of the hope research published in the past three decades. There have been less than 20 quantitative studies, not including studies using the Snyder Hope Scales, conducted about hope in a 16 year period: 1975-1991 (Farran, Herth, Popovich, 1995). The studies were conducted with the multiple scales that were first developed. None of the scales were used consistently over time. None of the previously created hope definitions, scales or research findings have come to the forefront as a leader (Snyder, 2000a; 2000b). Although the hope definitions have developed over time based on previous definitions the research on hope seems to be individual and not connected with the other work being completed in the area (Snyder, 2000a; 2000b).

Since the early 1980s, hope has been researched by many research groups in the psychology discipline using the Snyder Hope Scales. This field is more similar to social work and will be the focus of this literature review. This research has become more diverse in terms of populations and geographic locations, but specific attention has not been paid to potential variations in demographic characteristics such as gender. This research has been conducted using primarily the Snyder Hope Scales. Snyder has conducted the bulk of the research related to hope with colleagues and students (Farran, Herth, & Popovich, 1995).

Current areas of research related to hope theory are divided into 4 major sections: academic, athletic, physical well-being and psychological well-being. Research in each area has demonstrated positive results reporting scores indicating that higher hope is correlated with higher levels of performance, coping, mental well-being and physical health.

The State Hope Scale has been used to measure hope with homeless veterans being treated for substance abuse (Irving, Tefler, & Blake, 1997); college students (Snyder et al., 1996); and college athletes

(Curry, Snyder, Cook, Ruby, & Rehm, 1997). The State Hope Scale only considers a person's level of hope at one point of time and is based on her/his current situation.

On the other hand, the Trait Hope Scale considers the long standing hope a person regardless of the situation a person is currently experiencing. The Trait Hope Scale was first administered in 1985, with the results being published in 1988 (Harris, 1988). Since completion of the Trait Hope Scale, it has been used more often than other scales in the past 14 years with more than 15 studies in multiple populations.

Health psychology has given great consideration to the effects of trait hope on both primary prevention and secondary prevention. Primary prevention such as taking care of one's body through exercise, diet and regular check ups are considered to be factors aimed to reduce potential for illness. High trait hope people have been shown to follow these preventative measures more frequently than low hope people. Secondary prevention, directed at reducing a problem once it has appeared, includes things such as treatment compliance with medication and testing. Physical well-being studies have considered hope in people with chronic pain, cancer, diabetes, and asthma. Research results have indicated that high hope people are more inclined to have or learn coping skills for dealing with their illness and adhere to treatment plans. High hope people have also reported lower levels of distress related to their illness and fewer doctor visits.

Research results have indicated that performance in athletic competition is better depending on the competitor's level of trait hope. Research has been conducted with both males and females in university track competition. Results indicated that athletes with higher hope improved their success rate by 56% from the beginning of a season until the end. Research with girls in a summer camp for athletes reported that girls with higher levels of hope were less likely to think about quitting activities. One study conducted with athletes allowed for a group of students to participate in a course on hope. These athletes were followed for the next year. It was determined that they showed improvement after the course and were able to maintain their level of success. Research with athletes and hope is still in the early stages of investigation.

Areas of academic research have reported increased grade school achievement test scores and high school GPAs with increased hope. GPA level is also higher for college students with a higher level of trait hope. Snyder et al. (2000a; 2000b) reported that hope is predictive when controlling for IQ, self-esteem and previous grades. They reported that the predictivity of hope related to GPA was found after following

200 students (100 females/100 males) for 6 years. High hope students have a higher graduation rate than those who have lower levels of hope. Authors have correctly speculated that high hope teachers are more encouraging to students in reaching their goals. Hope scales have been positively correlated with teacher encouragement scales (r = .49) (Culver, 1992).

Hope in terms of psychological well-being has been tested with psychology students and inpatient psychiatric patients. Multiple authors have reported that high hope people have stronger and more attachments with other people therefore are less likely to be lonely like their low hope counterparts. High hope people indicated that they have the ability to call on friends for help when they need support. There are fewer reports of suicidal ideation and attempts among high hope people. High hope people reported being more inspired, energized and challenged by life. High hope people tend to learn from their past experiences and are more tolerant and forgiving of others. Research has also shown that people who have lost their parents to death or whose parents are divorced are more inclined to be low hope people.

Gaps in Research

Most of the original research was conducted in the medical field and has slowly moved into the social sciences. Research has been with limited populations (cancer, elderly, students, psychiatric patients) and other than the studies with students all results are based on people who are patients. Studies have become more diverse in the past 6 years although there has been almost no work that specifically compares different races or ages and little research considering gender differences. The research that has been performed in the social sciences has been with psychology students or psychiatric patients working with a psychologist. There is no research designed to compare hope in one person to that of another person based on characteristics of the individual or an environment in which the person exists.

There's a general lack of information and literature on hope or hope theory in the social work field. Research indicates that hope measurement tools are effective in other fields of studies with a variety of populations, but there is a need to look at hope with employees and more specifically with social service providers. Scales created to measure hope have never been used to assess hope in professionals or employees. They have not been applied to diverse social service client populations or social service providers.

There is a need to test the hope scales with social service providers to determine if they actually measure hope with this population. If the Snyder Trait Hope Scale model fits the context of social service providers well, there are many possible implications for developing interventions to increase levels of hope with social service providers and ultimately clients. Hope theory has not been considered in social work to date. None of the current scales have been used to determine if they, in fact, measure hope in the social services fields. Additionally, despite the work that has been done with hope in other fields there has not been any research conducted with professionals. It is possible that differences exist in service provider's strength based practice based on whether an organization employs hope based practices. Social work is a profession that would benefit from increased knowledge related to hope because of its focus on reaching goals for the well-being of clients.

To instill hope in others one must have a sense of their own hope. With the responsibility to better the well-being of clients bestowed upon the social work profession, it would present as an important endeavor to strive to learn about hope and how to assist people, both clients and providers, in gaining knowledge about assessing, nurturing and maintaining.

REFERENCES

Arches, J. (1991). Social structure, burnout, and job satisfaction. *Social Work, 36*, 202-206.

Averill, J.R., Catlin, G., & Chon, K.K. (1990). *Rules of Hope*. New York, NY: Springer-Verlag.

Barker, R.L. (1999). *The Social Work Dictionary (4th Edition)*. Baltimore, MD: NASW Press.

Beck, A.T., Kovacs, M., & Weissman, A. (1975). Hopelessness and suicidal behavior. *Journal of American Medical Association, 234*(11), 1146-1149.

Beck, C., Rawlins, R., & Williams, S. (1984). *Mental Health-Psychiatric Nursing: A Holistic Life Cycle Approach*. St. Louis, MO: C.V. Mosby.

Blankertz, L., & Robinson, S. (1996). Who is the psychosocial rehabilitation worker? *Psychiatric Rehabilitation Journal, 19*(4), 3-13.

Bloch, E. (1986). *The Principle of Hope*. Loudon, England: Basil Blackwell.

Braddock, D., & Mitchell, D. (1992). *Residential Services and Developmental Disabilities in the United States*. Edited by Michal J. Begab. Washington, D.C.: American Association on Mental Retardation.

Cherniss, C. (1980). *Staff Burnout: Job Stress in the Human Services*. Beverly Hills, CA: Sage Publications.

Chung, M.L. (1990). *Phenomenological nursing study on the critically ill patient's feelings of hopelessness.* Unpublished master's thesis, Ewha Woman's University, Seoul, South Korea.

Corcoran, K.J., & Bryce, A.K. (1983). Intervention in the experience of burnout: Effects of skill development. *Journal of Social Service Research, 7,* 71-79.

Cramer, K.M., & Dyrkacz, L. (1998). Differential prediction of maladjustment scores with the Snyder hope subscales. *Psychological Reports, 83,* 1035-1041.

Culver, N.F. (1992). *A validation of the encouragement scale-teacher form.* Unpublished doctoral dissertation, University of Georgia, Athens.

Curry, L.A., Snyder, C.R., Cooke, D.L., Ruby, B.C., & Rehm. M. (1997). The role of hope in student-athlete academic and sport achievement. *Journal of Personality and Social Psychology, 73,* 1257-1267.

Drake, B., & Yadama, G.N. (1996). A structural equation model of burnout and job exit among child protective services workers. *Social Work Research, 20*(3), 179-187.

Edelwich, J. (1980). *Burn-Out: Stages of Disillusionment in the Helping Professions.* New York, NY: Human Sciences Press.

Elliott, J.A. (2005). *Interdisciplinary Perspectives on Hope.* Hauppage, NY: Nova Science Publishers, Inc.

Erikson, E.H. (1982). *The Life Cycle Completed: A Review.* New York, NY: Norton.

Fahs Beck, D. (1987). Counselor burnout in family service agencies. *Social Casework, 68,* 3-15.

Farran, K.A., Herth, J., & Popovich, M. (1995). *Hope and Hopelessness: Critical Clinical Constructs.* Thousand Oaks, CA: Sage Publications.

Farran, K.A. & Popovich, J. (1990). Hope: A relevant concept for geriatric psychiatry. *Archives in Psychiatric Nursing, 4,* 127-130.

Frankl, V.E. (1992). *Man's Search for Meaning: An Introduction to Logotherapy (4th Edition).* Boston, MA: Beacon Press.

Frankl, V.E. (1963). *Man's Search for Meaning.* New York, NY: Washington Square.

Freudenberger, H.J., & Richelson, G. (1980). *Burnout: The High Cost of High Achievement.* Garden City, NY: Anchor Press.

Fromm, E. (1968). *The Revolution of Hope: Toward a Humanized Technology.* New York, NY: Harper and Row.

Geurts, S., Schaufeli, W., & De Jonge, J. (1998). Burnout and intention to leave among health-care professionals: A social psychological approach. *Journal of Social and Clinical Psychology, 1793,* 341-362.

Gibson, F., McGrath, A., & Reid, N. (1989). Occupational stress in social work. *British Journal of Social Work, 10,* 1-18.

Gottschalk, L. (1974). A hope scale applicable to verbal samples. *Archives of General Psychiatry, 30,* 779-785.

Grossart-Marticek, R., Kanazire, D.T., Better, H., & Schmidt, P. (1983). Psychosomatic factors involved in the process of cancerogenesis. *Psychotherapeutic Psychosomatics, 40,* 191-210.

Hagen, J.L. (1989). Income maintenance workers; Burned-out, dissatisfied, and leaving. *Journal of Social Service Research, 13,* 47-63.

Harris, C.D. (1988). *Hope: Construct definitions and the development of an individual differences scale.* Unpublished doctoral dissertation, Department of Psychology, University of Kansas, Lawrence.

Herth, K.A. (1991). Development and refinement of an instrument to measure hope. *Scholarly Inquiry for Nursing Practice, 5*(1), 39-51.

Himle, D.O., Jayaratne, S.D., & Thyness, P.A. (1986). Predictors of job satisfaction, burnout and turnover among social workers in Norway and the USA: A cross-cultural study. *International Social Work, 29*, 323-334.

Irving, L.M., Tefler, L., & Blake, D. (1997). Hope, coping, and social support in combat-related post-traumatic stress disorder. *Journal of Traumatic Stress, 10*, 463-477.

Itzhaky, H., & Lipschitz-Elhawi, R. (2004). Hope as a strategy in supervising social workers of terminally ill patients. *Health and Social Work, 29*(1), 46-54.

Jayaratne, S., & Chess, W.A. (1988). Dealing with work stress and strain: Is the perception of support more important than its use?" *Journal of Applied Behavioral Science, 24*, 191-202.

Jayaratne, S., & Chess, W.A. (1984). Job satisfaction, burnout, and turnover: A national study. *Social Work, 24*, 448-453.

Knapp, M., Harissis, K., & Missiakoulos, S. (1981). Who leaves social work? *The British Journal of Social Work, 11*, 421-444.

LeCroy, C.S., & Rank, M.R. (1986). Factors associated with burnout in the social services: An exploratory study. *Journal of Social Service Research, 10*, 23-39.

Maslach, C., & Jackson, S.E. (1981). The measurement of experienced burnout. *Journal of Occupational Behavior, 2*, 99-113.

Miller, J.F., & Powers, M. (1988). Development of an instrument to measure hope. *Nursing Research, 37*(1), 6-10.

Mor Barak, M.E., Nissly, J.A., & Levin, A. (2001). Antecedents to retention and turnover among child welfare, social work, and other human service employees: What can we learn from past research? A review and metanalysis. *Social Services Review, 74*(4), 625-660.

NASW. (1999). *Code of Ethics.* Baltimore, MD: NASW Press.

Nowotny, M. (1989). Assessment of hope in patients with cancer: Development of an instrument. *Oncology Nursing Forum, 16*(1), 75-79.

Owen, D. (1989). Nurses' perspectives on the meaning of hope in patients with cancer: A qualitative study. *Oncology Nursing Forum, 16*(1), 75-79.

Pines, A., Aronson, E., & Kafry, D. (1981). *Burnout: From Tedium to Personal Growth.* New York, NY: Free Press.

Pines, A., & Kafry, D. (1978). Occupational tedium in the social services. *Social Work, 23*, 499-507.

Richter, C.P. (1957). On the phenomenon of sudden death in animals and man. *Psychosomatic Medicine, 19*(3), 191-198.

Schmale, A.H. (1964). A genetic view of affects: With specific reference to the genesis of helplessness and hopelessness. *Psychoanalytic Study of the Child, 19*, 287-310.

Snyder, C.R. (2002). Hope theory: Rainbows in the mind. *Psychological Inquiry, 13*(4), 249-275.

Snyder, C.R. (Ed.) (2000a). *Handbook of Hope: Theory, Measures, and Applications.* San Diego, CA: Academic Press.

Snyder, C.R. (2000b). The past and future of hope. *Journal of Social and Clinical Psychology, 19*, 11-28.

Snyder, C.R. (1998). Hope. In H.S. Friedman (Ed.), *Encyclopedia of Mental Health* (pp. 421-431). San Diego, CA: Academic.

Snyder, C.R. (1994a). *The Psychology of hope: You Can Get There From Here.* New York, NY: Free Press.

Snyder, C.R. (1994b). Hope, goal blocking thoughts, and test-related anxieties. *Psychological Reports, 84,* 206-206.

Snyder, C.R. (1989). Reality negotiation: From excuses to hope and beyond. *Journal of Social and Clinical Psychology, 8,* 130-157.

Snyder, C.R., Harris, C., Anderson, J.R., Holleran, S.A., Irving, L.M., Sigmon, S.T., Yoshinobu, L., Gibb, J., Langelle, C., & Harney, P. (1991). The will and the ways: Development and validation of an individual differences measure of hope. *Journal of Personality and Social Psychology, 60,* 570-585.

Snyder, C.R., Sympson, S.C., Ybasco, F.C., Borders, T.F., Babyak, M.A., & Higgins, R.L. (1996). Development and validation of the State Hope Scale. *Journal of Personality and Social Psychology, 2,* 321-335.

Snyder, C.R., Irving, L., & Anderson, J.R. (1991). Hope and health: Measuring the wills and the ways. In C.R. Snyder & D.R. Forsyth (Eds.), *Handbook of Social and Clinical Psychology: The Health Perspective* (p. 285-305). Elmsford, NY: Pergamon Press.

Soderfeldt, M., Soderfeldt, B., & Warg, L. (1995). Burnout in social work. *Social Work, 40*(5), 639-646.

Sowers-Hoag, K.M., & Thyer, B.A. (1987). Burnout among social work professional: A behavioral approach to causal and interventive knowledge. *Journal of Sociology and Social Welfare, 14*(3), 105-118.

Staudt, M., Howard, M.O., & Drake, B. (2001). The operationalization, implementation, and effectiveness of the strengths perspective: A review of empirical studies. *Journal of Social Service Review, 27*(3), 1-21.

Stotland, E. (1969). *The Psychology of Hope.* San Francisco, CA: Jossey-Bass.

Streepy, J. (1981). Direct-service providers and burnout. *Social Casework, 62,* 352-361.

Sumerlin, J. (1997). Self-actualization and hope. *Journal of Social Behavior and Personality, 12,* 1101-1110.

Walsh, J.A. (1987). Burnout and values in the social services profession. *Social Casework: Journal of Contemporary Social Work, May,* 279-283.

Weick, A., Rapp, C., Sullivan, W.P., & Kisthardt, W. (1989). A strengths perspective for social work practice. *Social Work, July,* 350-354.

doi:10.1300/J137v15n04_07

Reinforcing the Divide:
The Influence of the U.S. Census
on American Identity Development

John W. Miller, Jr.

SUMMARY. Accounts of race in the United States have traditionally been steeped in prejudicial notions consistent with the society (Lusane, 2000; U.S. Census Bureau, 2000; Griffin, Caplinger, Lively, Malcom, McDaniel, & Nelsen, 1997). The U.S. Census has been used as an instrument in the continued dichotomous division of American citizens into either one of two groups, Whites and Nonwhites (Ngai, 1999). This essay examines the impact of the U.S. Census on U.S. law, public policy, and distribution of privilege between Whites and Nonwhites. This essay also addresses the influence of census-based racial classification on social work practice and education. doi:10.1300/J137v15n04_08 *[Article copies available for a fee from The Haworth Document Delivery Service: 1-800-HAWORTH. E-mail address: <docdelivery@haworthpress.com> Website: <http://www.HaworthPress. com> © 2007 by The Haworth Press, Inc. All rights reserved.]*

KEYWORDS. Census, race, hyphenated-American, social work

John W. Miller, Jr., MSW, is a Doctoral Student, University of Tennessee, College of Social Work (E-mail: Jmille44@utk.edu).

[Haworth co-indexing entry note]: "Reinforcing the Divide: The Influence of the U.S. Census on American Identity Development." Miller, John W. Jr. Co-published simultaneously in *Journal of Human Behavior in the Social Environment* (The Haworth Press, Inc.) Vol. 15, No. 4, 2007, pp. 125-141; and: *Adult Development and Well-Being: The Impact of Institutional Environments* (ed: Catherine N. Dulmus, and Karen M. Sowers) The Haworth Press, 2007, pp. 125-141. Single or multiple copies of this article are available for a fee from The Haworth Document Delivery Service [1-800-HAWORTH, 9:00 a.m. - 5:00 p.m. (EST). E-mail address: docdelivery@haworthpress.com].

INTRODUCTION

Our historical records reflect the racial prejudices of the times in which they were created, and consequently as a historical record, the census is embedded with our culture's racism (Lusane, 2000; U.S. Census Bureau, 2000; Griffin, Caplinger, Lively, Malcom, McDaniel, & Nelsen, 1997). The first U.S. Census was taken in 1790 (U.S. Census, 2000), and since then there have been many important changes in the philosophy, legislation, and priority of social relations within American society and law. Although significant changes have occurred, the dichotomous relationship between the classification of White and nonwhite American citizens is as present currently as it was in 1790. As an important social institution, the U.S. Census has continued the dichotomous division of American citizens into one of two groups, Whites and nonwhites (Ngai, 1999).

This dichotomous racial relationship is disempowering to U.S. minorities, and the continuation of policy, through the U.S. Census Bureau's via its current classification system, perpetuates a class hierarchy and should be addressed by scholars.

> The census is a generally unacknowledged critical actor in the nation's racialization process. Race construction occurs from many social vectors and one must be careful never to overly determine one particular site. Popular culture, historical experiences, institutional socialization, and many other variables, operating at different levels of intensity and influence, contribute to the process. (Lusane, 2000, p. 155)

Thus, if institutions are to be thought of as dominant mechanisms for control managed by human actors who are seeking some type of status quo, some state of just being, the census becomes both the framework for managing (by determining the categories, etc.) while also serving as the mechanism that educates us as to what we are (or aren't). Like many other American institutions (i.e., education, religion, law, etc.) the U.S. Census' influence on U.S. citizens today cannot be separated from the parameters (i.e., racism, classism) that surrounded its creation.

In this article I will first provide an overview of the historical and social context in which the foundation of the U.S. Census was developed. I trace the movement of the Census from different government organizations, and examine the original classifications of people that were and were not counted by the first Census. This is done to decipher what effect the social context of the first Census has had on reinforcing the divide between Whites and nonwhites. Also, I examined the significance of the development of Census classification criteria.

Central to this study is the historical context surrounding the evolution of the Census classification of White. I argue that over time, the classification White has transformed, from simply a racial category to a racial and ethnic group. Public policies such as the Immigration Act of 1924 further influenced Census classification criteria and created an ideology of the hyphenated American. The Census has been a strong institutional force in influencing U.S. governmental policies for counting, and undercounting citizens. In this essay, I also highlight related policies such as the *Standards for Maintaining, Collecting, and Presenting Federal Data on Race*, and argue that these measures have been ineffective in addressing the racial hierarchy created by the Census and similar measures.

This article argues that the dichotomous relationship between White and Nonwhite American citizenship perpetuated by Census classification has bearings on every American citizen. The hierarchical implication of a natural White ownership of American citizenship has negative consequences on many aspects of everyday life. The field of social work has neglected to address the institutional impact of the racial classification divide, created and maintained by the U.S. Census, on all Americans.

HISTORY OF RACIAL CLASSIFICATION IN THE U.S. CENSUS

A nationwide population census taken on a regular basis dates from the establishment of the United States. Article I, Section 2, of the United States Constitution required that,

> Representatives and direct taxes shall be apportioned among the several states which may be included within this union, according to their respective numbers, which shall be determined by adding to the whole number of free persons, including those bound to service for a term of years, and excluding Indians not taxed, three-fifths of all other persons. The actual Enumeration shall be made within three Years after the first Meeting of the Congress of the United States, and within every subsequent term of ten years, in such manner as they shall by law direct. (U.S. Constitution)

All other persons included mainly slaves and suggested that to establish representation in the House of Representatives, free men were counted as one person, and slaves were counted as three-fifths of a person (U.S. Census, 2002). The agreed upon language of the U.S. Constitution was the result of The Great Compromise (Hodgkinson, 1995). The Great Compromise dealt with the representation, congressionally, of how to count slaves in a very subtle way. Representatives from the North realized that southern leaders would demand some counting of slaves in determining the representation of a state. Few southern leaders, however, had the gall to claim that slaves, who could not vote, should be counted the same as free people. The leaders decided that all free persons, excluding and those Europeans bound to service, would count as citizens for the purposes of representation in the House (Zinn, 2003; Hodgkinson, 1995). "All other persons," however, such as slaves, counted three-fifths, and "Indians not taxed" were not counted at all. The three-fifths compromise was adopted without much controversy and set the tone for the separation of Whites from nonwhites (Zinn, 2003).

Race as a Significant Social Category

In 1790 it was clear that many slaves had lighter skins than their masters, so to increase the size of the slave population, the "one drop of blood" rule appeared (Hodgkinson, 1995). The one-drop rule signaled that just one drop of Black blood defined a person as Black (Strain, 2003). Therefore any child of a slave and slave-owner was considered eligible for slavery. Over time, this enlarged the slave pool considerably. Prior to the arrival of slaves, colonists classified themselves by numerous criteria, but not race. Instead; class, family name, wealth, heritage, education, religious preference, and community of origin were used as the prominent indicators of division amongst the ranks of colonists (Zinn, 2003). Arguably, there is a strong correlation between the onset of race as a significant classification criterion and the arrival of Black slaves into the U.S. during the mid to late seventeenth century.

Although indentured servants from Europe had been working off their debts and crimes in English colonies for decades, the use of skin color to make distinctions amongst persons reflects the increasingly tenuous state of race relations during the mid to late seventeenth century (Strain, 2003). This ideology of color implied that White colonists and future Americans, regardless of any status or circumstance, were naturally superior to Blacks (Strain, 2003). The U.S. Constitution further legitimized this ideology by classifying all Blacks as only three-fifths of a

White person in the eyes of the government. Mainstream social psychology holds that prejudice and racism begin with false generalizations (Gaines & Reed, 1995). The false generalizations that influenced the development of the foundation of *race* relations within the United States have had trickle down effects. These influences have not just affected the lives of Blacks, or African Americans, but every other hyphenated American as well.

The Development of the Hyphenated-American

The concept of the hyphenated American can be traced back to several important legislative acts that addressed immigration policy. The Nationality Act of 1790 was the first public policy to exclusively reserve American citizenship for Whites only. It provided the basis excluding African, Chinese, Japanese, Filipino, Asian Indian, and Korean immigrants from citizenship (Ngin, 1993). The Nationality Act of 1870 further encoded racial prerequisites to citizenship by establishing the familiar U.S. Census classifications of Black and White (Tibor, 1995). The act had bearings on the creation of the Chinese Exclusion Act of 1882, which declared Chinese immigrants ineligible for citizenship by implying that since Chinese immigrants were not White, they could not become naturalized citizens (Yamashita & Park, 1985; Zinn, 2003; Ngai, 2003). The law, however, was unclear about the citizenship status of other future hyphenated Americans who would immigrate to the U.S., from Mexico, Japan, Syria, etc., in the late nineteenth and twentieth centuries. Between 1887 and 1923 the federal courts heard twenty-five cases challenging the racial prerequisite to citizenship, which reflected a growing dissatisfaction with racial classification in minority communities (Hamm, 1999). Rather than being used as an instrument to remedy this dissatisfaction, the U.S. Census became an institutional force that influenced immigration policy in increasingly restrictive ways for minorities.

The Immigration Act of 1924 restricted immigration to 150,000 new immigrants a year based on quotas formed largely in part by the U.S. Census (Ngai, 1999). The Quota Board was developed to set immigration quotas using Census racial categories to make its calculations, and in the census's racial criteria all Blacks and mulattoes were omitted from the population of the U.S. In 1920, Blacks accounted for approximately 9 percent (13,000) of the total U.S. population. Had they been included in the base population governing the quotas, the African nations from which they originated would have received 9 percent of the total immigration quota (Ngai, 1999). Since the Black and *mulatto* populations were omitted in the calculation of the quota quotient, the 13,000 slots that should have gone to African nations were added to the quota total for European nations. As a result, the Census became the basis not only for institutional counting, but also for regulating the presence of nonwhites in the United States.

An additional significant problem that arose from the development of the Immigration Act was the evolution of "national-origin" (Ngai, 1999). "The central theme of the legislative process that led to the passage of the law was that of a race-based nativism that favored the Nordics of northern and western Europe over the undesirable races of eastern and southern Europe" (Ngai, 1999, p. 2). The Immigration Act compromised racial categories on two levels. First, the Immigration Act differentiated Europeans according to nationality and thus ranked them in a hierarchy of desirability, i.e., Irish vs. British, or Jewish vs. Christian. Second, the Immigration Act created a White American race in which all persons of European descent shared a common "whiteness" that made them distinct from the nonwhites. European-Americans simultaneously acquired two identities, and an ethnicity based on national identity as well as a racial identity based on *whiteness* presumed to be unchangeable (Ngai, 1999).

Non-European immigrants, Japanese, Chinese, Mexicans, and Filipinos, however, acquired ethnic and racial identities that were one and the same, which forever rendered them "foreign" to the nation. Analysis of the Immigration Act of 1924 (Ngai, 1999, 2003; Hamm, 1999; Tibor, 1995) suggests that immigration law and policy were deeply implicated in a broader racial and ethnic remapping of the nation during the 1920s. This remapping took place in mutually constituting realms of demography, economics, and law (Franco, 1985). Subsequent changes in immigration patterns and policy included: the migration of African Americans from the South to northern cities and the legal justification for de facto segregation in the North, and the completion of the legal process of forced assimilation of American Indians (Ngai, 2003).

The Role of the Census

The government of United States established laws, such as, Article I, Section 2, of the United States Constitution, The Nationality Acts of 1790 & 1870, and The Immigration Act of 1924, that implied that true American citizenship belonged to *Whites* only. The institution of the U.S. Census has served as the governmental vehicle to do more than just enumerate its citizens, but also to promote a class hierarchy that dichotomously separated its citizens into the two groups of *White* or *nonwhite*. The Census established this dichotomy in 1790 by counting only free Whites (U.S. Census Bureau, 2002). A racial divide was further promoted by the use of Census data to classify citizens as *Black, mulatto, quadroon,* and *octoroon* on the basis of the *one-drop* rule (Nguyen, 1996; Lusane, 2000; Green & Manzi, 2002). Multiple labeling practices for nonwhites lead to the development of *hyphenated* American citizenship (Ngin, 1993; Ngai, 1999, 2003). "There is not a country in world history in which racism has been more important, for a long time, as the United States" (Zinn, 2003, p. 23). Throughout the late nineteenth and early to mid-twentieth century, a tumultuous period in American race relations, the classification of White was given superior status to other classifications of American citizenship by claiming race as well as ethnic status (Griffen et al., 1997; Ngai, 1999). U.S. nation building was configured in decisive ways around the debates regarding slavery, the race issue, and the distribution of economic power (Zinn, 2003; Griffen et al., 1997; Lusane, 2000). "State intervention into these discourses, including the political, and racial, use of the Census, was conscious and deliberate" (Lusane, 1999, p. 155). Griffen et al. (1997) found that the definition of populations, White, Black, octoroon, quadroon, Indian, etc., was a major factor in the passing of laws that amended or rewrote state constitutions to the benefit of Whites during the late nineteenth and early twentieth centuries. Thus, the U.S. Census served as the governing institution of American social hierarchy and its continual use of racial labeling has had a significant institutional impact on the identity development of nonwhites.

"In nearly every Census since 1790, race has been defined differently, and the inclusion or exclusion of any specific racial group has been contingent on the confluence of the political imperatives of the moment and balance of power between various social actors" (Lusane, 1999, p. 155). The Census has always been a site of racial contention, and no instance of census taking has been free of the political, social, and ideological issues that affect the politics of a nation. Thus, the way the U.S. has classified and enumerated its citizens has changed between almost every decennial Census since 1790 (see Table 1). Although each of the various classifications of nonwhites has been altered over the 214-year period since the first Census, the classification White has been unmolested (Lee, 1993). "The decision to fashion the nation, in part via the Census, as "White" was an elite one, albeit supported by a White popular consensus" (Lusane, 1999, p. 155). Political and racial undertones informed and influenced the first Census and every one since then

TABLE 1. Historical Overview of Changing Racial Classifications on the U.S. Census Form 1870-2000

Year	Classifications
1870	White, Black, Indian
1880	White, Black, Indian
1890	White, Black, Mulatto, Quadroon, Octoroon, Indian, Chinese, Japanese
1900	White, Black, Indian, Chinese, Japanese
1910	White, Black, Indian, Chinese, Japanese, Other
1920	White, Black, Indian, Chinese, Japanese, Other
1930	White, Negro, Mexican, Indian, Chinese, Japanese, Filipino, Hindu, Korean, Other
1940	White, Negro, Indian, Chinese, Japanese, Filipino, Hindu, Korean, Other
1950	White, Negro, American Indian, Chinese, Japanese, Filipino, Other
1960	White, Negro, American Indian, Chinese, Japanese, Filipino, Hawaiian, Part Hawaiian, Aleut, Eskimo, Other, etc.
1970	White, Negro or Black, Indian (American), Chinese, Japanese, Filipino, Hawaiian, Korean, Other
1980	White, Black or Negro, Indian (American), Chinese, Japanese, Filipino, Vietnamese, Asian Indian, Hawaiian, Guamanian, Samoan, Eskimo, Aleut, Other
1990	White, Black or Negro, Indian (American), Eskimo, Aleut, Asian or Pacific Islander, Chinese, Japanese, Filipino, Hawaiian, Korean, Vietnamese, Asian Indian, Samoan, Guamanian, Other
2000	White, Black, African American or Negro, American Indian or Alaska Native, Asian Indian, Japanese, Native Hawaiian, Chinese, Korean, Guamanian or Chomorro, Filipino, Vietnamese, Samoan, Other Asian, Other Pacific Islander

Source. U.S. Census Bureau, Measuring America: The Decennial Censuses from 1790 to 2000.

(Ngai, 2003; Ngin, 1993; Lusane, 2000; Hodgkinson, 1995). Therefore, withstanding centuries of political regime change, the institutional impact of the divisive nature of the Census remains the same. Despite specific categorization changes from time to time, America is just as divided by the Census today (White, Nonwhite) as it was back in 1790.

U.S. GOVERNMENT STANDARDS ON RACE CLASSIFICATION

Statistical Policy Directive No. 15

In 1977, the Federal Interagency of Committee on Education (FICE) developed standards on how federal government agencies would classify citizens. The Office of Management and Budget (OMB), which houses the Census Bureau, adopted the FICE recommendations and called the new classification regulation Statistical Policy Directive No. 15

(U.S. Census Bureau, 1997). The standards were developed to provide consistent and comparable data on race and ethnicity throughout the Federal government for various of statistical and administrative programs (U.S. Census Bureau, 1995, 1997, 2000, 2002). The standard set by Statistical Policy Directive No. 15 set four categories for data on race, which were Hispanic Origin American Indian or Alaska Native, Asian or Pacific Islander, Black, and White.

Data collected from Statistical Policy Directive No. 15 was needed to monitor equal access to housing, education, employment opportunities, etc. for population groups that historically had experienced discrimination and differential treatment because of their race or ethnicity (U.S. Census Bureau, 1997). These categories represented a socio-political construct designed to organize data collection data on race and ethnicity, and lacked any anthropological or scientific basis. The standards were set not only for the decennial censuses, but also for school registration and mortgage lending applications (U.S. Census Bureau, 1997), indicating the broad reaching influence of the OMB classifications in the lives of American citizens.

The standard set forth by the OMB via Statistical Policy Directive No. 15 drew criticism because it ignored the increasing racial and ethnic diversity of the U.S. (U.S. Census Bureau, 1995; Hodgkinson, 1995; Johnson, 1994). Another major criticism of the directive was that since it was used for civil right enforcement and program administration, many groups of people who did not categorize themselves as any of the five groups presented by the OMB were at risk of being discriminated against (U.S. Census Bureau, 1997). It was also criticized for the influence it had on the undercounting of persons due to not having exhausted the racial/ethnic categories that were to be chosen from (U.S. Census Bureau, 1995; Lusane, 2000).

Standards for Maintaining, Collecting, and Presenting Federal Data on Race and Ethnicity

In response to criticisms, OMB announced in July 1993 that it would undertake a comprehensive review of the categories set in place by Statistical Policy Directive No. 15 (U.S. Census Bureau, 1997). The Interagency Committee for the Review of the Racial and Ethnic Standards (ICRRES) was formed to facilitate the participation of federal agencies in the review. ICRRES was composed of over thirty federal agencies that "represented the many and diverse Federal needs for data on race and ethnicity, including statutory requirements for such data" (U.S.

Census Bureau, 1997, p. 2). The review's objective was to enhance the accuracy of the demographic information collected by the federal government. ICRRES addressed the various criticisms, considered suggestions for changing the current categories, and developed a research agenda for what they deemed to be the most significant issues.

Issues ICRRES investigated included the collection and classification of data on persons that identified themselves as *multiracial*; combining the concepts of race, ethnicity, and ancestry; changing the terminology used for particular categories; and adding new categories to the current minimum set (U.S. Census Bureau, 1997, 2002; Gibson & Young, 2002). ICRRES conducted several surveys and interviews, including the 1996 National Content Survey (NCS), and the 1996 Race and Ethnic Targeted Test (RAETT). These surveys were designed to answer some of the criticisms the previous directive drew. ICRRES generated questions on the NCS and RAETT from findings of an internal review in which ICRRES compiled a list of possible questions that may have been of interest to American citizens (U.S. Census Bureau, 1997). The questions NCS and RAETT investigated included: Should a *multiracial* category be added so that respondents would not be forced to deny part of their heritage by having to choose a single category? Should an *"other"* category be added for individuals of multiracial heritage? Should the term *Black* be changed to African American? Should the American Indian or Alaska Native category be changed to Native American? Should Hispanic be moved into a racial category away from an ethnic classification? Should the name Hispanic be changed to Latino? Should Middle Eastern or Arab, and Cape Verdean be ethnic categories? Should Native Hawaiian be made a separate category or included into the Alaskan Native, American Indian, Asian, or Pacific Islander category (U.S. Census Bureau, 1997). Absent from the question list was any question that considered expanding the Census category "White."

For each of the proposed questions, the findings were tabulated, and then ICRRES used the results to help determine the new standard that federal governmental agencies would be held to. The new standard was named the Standards for Maintaining, Collecting, and Presenting Federal Data on Race and Ethnicity. Although the purpose of ICRRES was to make racial categories more exhaustive, ICRRES did not speculate any regarding how Whites would like to be classified, thereby maintaining the White/nonwhite dichotomy. The fact that "whiteness" went without revision is astonishing as at least one member of the ICRRES committee, the U.S. Department of Labor and the Bureau of Labor Statistics (BLS), had previously found a need to revisit the category.

In 1995 the Bureau of Labor and Statistics compiled a report, *A CPS Supplement for Testing Methods of Collecting Racial and Ethnic Information,* which surveyed Americans' preferences of racial and ethnic terminology. The report examined each of the five previous classifications designated by Statistical Policy Directive No. 15. The results revealed a comparable amount of discrepancy regarding racial terminology preference amongst Whites and the other racial/ethnic classifications–Hispanic, Black, and American Indian (See Table 2).

The survey found that 38.7 percent of Whites preferred to be classified as something other than White or had no preference. Most Blacks

TABLE 2. Preference for Racial and Ethnic Terminology: May 1995

Preferred Terminology	Percent	Preferred Term	Percent
Hispanic		**White**	
Hispanic	57.9%	White	61.7%
Latino	11.8%	Caucasian	16.5%
Of Spanish Origin	12.3%	European American	2.4%
Some Other Term	7.9%	Anglo	1.0%
No preference	10.2%	Some other term	2.0%
		No preference	16.6%
Black		**American Indian**	
Black	44.2%	American Indian	49.8%
African American	28.1%	Alaskan Native	3.5%
Afro-American	12.1%	Native American	37.4%
Negro	3.3%	Some other term	3.7%
Colored	1.1%	No preference	5.7%
No preference	9.1%		
Multiracial			
Multiracial	28.4%		
More than one race	6.0%		
Biracial	5.7%		
Mixed race	16.0%		
Mestizo or Mestiza	2.3%		
Some other term	13.9%		
No preference	27.8%		

Source. Bureau of Labor Statistics, U.S. Department of Labor, *A CPS Supplement for Testing Methods of Collecting Racial and Ethnic Information: May 1995.*

(53.3 percent) surveyed preferred to be classified as Black or had no preference. Most Hispanics (70.1 percent) surveyed preferred to be classified as Hispanic or had no preference. A large majority of American Indians (87.6 percent) preferred to be called either American Indian or Native American. The study also addressed the proposed *multiracial* category and found that 56.2 percent of individuals that classified themselves as multiracial preferred either multiracial as a classification or had no preference (U.S. Bureau of Labor Statistics, 1995). With the BLS serving as a member of ICRRES, the lack of any questions regarding how Whites should have been classified within the *Standards for Maintaining, Collecting, and Presenting Federal Data on Race and Ethnicity* raises concern on several levels. First, without questioning Whites on either the NCS or RAETT of their racial preference, it may be implicitly suggested that the status of White is exclusive in its American ownership. Also, by only asking nonwhites their preferences to create a new set of standards, ICRRES was flawed in their data collection methods.

What ICRRES did by only asking nonwhites what they would like to be classified as was to fall victim to single source bias. The single source in this instance is nonwhites, therefore the new *Standards for Maintaining, Collecting, and Presenting Federal Data on Race and Ethnicity* are flawed. Without offering Whites the same opportunity offered to nonwhites to express their classification preference statistics on the 38.7 percent of Whites who do not prefer to be identified as White are in jeopardy of never being gathered and analyzed by federal government agencies. By continuing the exclusivity of White as the only classification without alternatives, ICRRES and OMB (and consequently the Census) further promoted the ideology that *whiteness* was mutually exclusive to American and was therefore both an ethnicity and race.

IMPLICATIONS

Social Welfare

The dichotomous relationship between *whites* and *nonwhites* asserted by the Census influences the social welfare of Americans in many ways. The racial differential in the Census undercount has become an important political subject, in the last two decades particularly, because Census undercounts directly affects political representation and federal resource distribution (Myers, 1992; Petersen, 1987). Since the first U.S. Census taken in 1790, there have been many important changes in the philosophy, legislation, and priority of social relations within American society through legislation such as the 1964 Civil Rights Act, and the 1965 Voting Rights Act (U.S. Census, 2000; Hoy, 2002).

Despite such changes, the dichotomous relationship between the classification of *White* and non*white* persons has only increased since 1790, and should not remain unchallenged. U.S. Census data is used to determine funding, enforcement, and eligibility for many federal programs that address access to voting rights, bilingual education, equal employment opportunities, energy assistance, lending practices, child assistance, aid to the elderly and handicapped, transportation projects, low-cost housing, and other areas of service (Hoy, 2002; Thomas & Hughes, 1986; U.S. Census Bureau, 1988; Nagda & Gutierrez, 2000). The field of Social Work has gone far too long without challenging these potential effects of institutionalized racism within the Census and its impact on the daily lives of all American citizens.

Social Work Education and Practice

"National demographic changes with increasing social diversity, and a rise in racial, ethnic, gender and other group-based tensions have posed special challenges for human service organizations" (Nagata & Gutierrez, 2000, p. 43). Because of this it is paramount that social workers continue to add to the state of the art as it pertains to the topic of social inequality via race relations in America. Empowerment theorists have argued that empowerment itself takes on multiple forms across people, shifts over time, and is based in several different contexts based on the person in the environment (Foster-Fishman, Salem, Chibnall, Legler, & Yapchai, 1998; Zimmerman, 1990, 1995).

With regard to the link between the legacy of the White/Nonwhite dichotomous breakdown of the Census and empowerment, I argue that the two will forever be closely associated due to a shared history. The history of the U.S. is filled with incidences in which the White majority has protected its claim to *true American* ownership (Zinn, 2003) via government mandates, laws and policies such as those discussed here, Article I, Section 2 of the U.S. Constitution, the Nationality Act of 1790, original Census enumeration tactics, the *one-drop rule*, the Immigration Act of 1922, etc. (U.S. Census, 2000; Ngai, 1999; Lusane, 2000; U.S. Constitution). This has been done both overtly, through laws and regulations, and covertly, by practices such as ignoring of BLS's racial preference survey (U.S. Census Bureau, 2000; Gibson & Jung, 2002; Nguyen, 1996; Lusane, 2000; Lee, 1993).

Ultimately, the division of American citizens into groups of Whites and Nonwhites is disempowering to both groups. "Empowerment refers to the process of gaining influence over events and outcomes of importance to an individual or group" (Foster-Fishman et al., 1998, p. 508). Nonwhites are disempowered through this empowerment perspective because of their lack of influence gained over time. When the dividing lines between superiority and inferiority (via the dichotomous racial categorization of the Census) still exist that were present in the year of the first Census (1790), nonwhites may feel disempowered because of the lack of change over the course of 215 years.

The official *Standards for Maintaining, Collecting, and Presenting Federal Data on Race and Ethnicity* guidelines reinforce the notion that nonwhites are not as empowered as Whites. By failing to question the appropriateness of suggesting alternative racial categories for all American citizens except Whites (U.S. Census Bureau, 1997; Lusane, 2000), the Standards reiterate the distinction between Whites and Nonwhites. This is also underscored by the lack of a homogenous Census racial classification system in which all Americans are classified as *hyphenated* Americans or not. Despite evidence (U.S. Bureau of Labor and Statistics, 1996) that there is no consensus amongst all racially classified groups in America of one unified racial classification preference over another, the continued separation and implied elitist nature of the separation of *Whites* and *Nonwhites* is a problem that social workers need to address.

> The "divided social world has profound implications for *Whites* as well as *Blacks* and for overt racists as well as those who are not. Most social psychologist seem to assume that a person's identification with particular groups is self-consistent. For example, a *White* male of Jewish heritage can and often does identify with those three groupings and also with being an American. But for an African American, identification as an American flies in the face of the all too real rift in American society." (Gaines & Reed, 1995, p. 99)

Social work educators and practitioners should be mindful of all of the possible influences of a divide between Whites and Nonwhites in the U.S. Census. "A great deal of what it means to be a *Black* is based on the assumptions, attitudes, and expectancies of *White* Americans" (Gaines

& Reed, 1995, p. 99). The profession of social work can do a better job of addressing the concerns of nonwhites by being more culturally sensitive.

> Being culturally aware is only a first step in addressing racism. However, it is insufficient in addressing the issues identified in this review. Minorities live with realities of poverty, a lack of resources, and racism that individual adaptation and social worker sensitivity alone cannot address. Although one can empower clients through individual intervention to take charge of their unique circumstances, realistically, clients alone do not have the resources to influence the kind of macro-level change required to address racism. Social work, by adopting an individualistic approach, tends to blame the victim while ignoring the ecological perspective and person-in-environment configuration. It gives lip service to fighting conditions of poverty, institutional practices that perpetuate racism, and other conditions external to the individual. (McMahon & Allen-Meares, 1992, p. 537)

By failing to have more research focused on the impact of broader social institutions on the lives on minorities, the field of Social Work is missing out on a great opportunity to be at the fore-front of new research. This proposed new research can address micro as well as macro-level concerns given the broad scope of social welfare issues that social workers address. Almost every area of concern that many social workers investigate (i.e., the homeless, foster care, juvenile justice, fair public housing practices, etc.) has been influenced by an overriding social institution. The effects of the social institution that is the U.S. Census should not be omitted from further scrutiny and investigation.

REFERENCES

Alonso, W. & Starr, P. (Eds.) (1987). The Politics of Numbers. New York: Russell Sage.

American Psychological Association (2002). Publication manual of the american psychological association (5th ed.). Washington, DC: Author.

Foster-Fishman, P.G., Salem, D.A., Chibnall, R.L., Leigler, L., & Yapchai, C. (1998). Empirical support for the critical assumptions of empowerment theory. *American Journal of Community Psychology, 26*(4), 507-537.

Franco, J. (1985). Intelligence test and social policy. *Journal of Counseling and Development, 64*, 278-279

Gaines, S. & Reed, E. (1995). Prejudice: From alport to dubois. *American Psychologist, 50*(2), 96-103.

Gibson, C. & Jung, K. (2002, September). Historical census statistics on population totals by race, 1790 to 1990, and by Hispanic origin, 1970-1990, for the United States, regions, divisions, and states (Working Paper Series No. 56). Retrieved January 26, 2004, from U.S. Census Bureau Reports Online: http://www.census.gov/population/www/documentation/twps0056.html.

Green, R. & Manzi, R. (2002). A comparison of methodologies for uncovering the structure of racial stereotype subgrouping. *Social Behavior and Personality, 30*(7), 709-728.

Griffin, L., Caplinger, C., Lively, K., Malcom, N., McDaniel, D., & Nelsen, C. (1997). Comparative-historical analysis and scientific inference: Disfranchisement in the U.S. south as a test case. *Historical Methods, 30*(1), 13-26.

Hamm, B. (1999). Redefining racism: Newspaper justification for the 1924 exclusion of japanese immigrants. *American Journalism, 16*(3), 53-69.

Hodgkinson, H. (1995). What should we call people? *Phi Delta Kappan, 77*(2), 173-179.

Hoy, S. (2000). Interpreting equal protection: Congress, the court, and the civil rights acts. *Journal of Law & Politics 2000, 16*(2), 381-478.

Johnson, A. (1994). *American government: People, institutions, and policies.* New York: Houghton Mifflin.

Johnson, M.P. & Roak, J.L. (1984). Black masters. A family of color in the old south. New York: Norton

Lee, S. M. (1993). Racial classifications in the us census: 1890-1990. *Ethnic and Racial Studies, 19*(1), 75-94.

Logan, R. & Cohen, I. (1970). The american Negro. New York: Houghton and Mifflin.

Lusane, C. (2000). Black no more: Race construction and the 2000 census. *National Political Science Review 2000, 8*, 151-170.

McMahon, A. & Allen-Meares, P. (1992). Is social work racist? A content analysis of recent literature [Electronic version]. 37(6), 533-539.

Myers, D. (1992). *Analysis with local census data: Portraits of change.* Boston, MA: Academic Press.

Nagda, B.A. & Gutierrez, L.M. (2000). A praxis and research agenda for multicultural human services organizations. *International Journal of Social Welfare, 9*, 43-53.

Ngai, M.M. (1999). The architecture of race in american immigration law: A reexamination of the immigration act of 1924. *The Journal of American History, 89*(1). Retrieved January 26, 2004, from Expanded Academic ASAP database.

Ngai, M.M. (2003). The strange career of the illegal alien: Immigration restriction and deportation policy in the united states, 1921-1965. *Law and History Review, 21*(1), 69-107.

Ngin, C. (1993). A new look at the old *race* language: Rethinking *race* and exclusion in social policy. *Explorations in Ethnic Studies, 16*(1), 5-18.

Nguyen, P. (1996). Census undercount and the undercount of the black population. *Western Journal of Black Studies, 20*(2), 96-103.

Strain, T. (Director). (2003). Race: The power of an illusion [Film]. California Newsreel Corporation.

Thomas, M., & Hughes, M. (1986). The continuing significance of race, class, and quality of life in America, 1972-1985 [Electronic version]. *American Sociological Review, 51*(6), 830-841.

Tibor, F. (1995). From nativism to the quota laws: Restrictionist pressure groups and the US congress 1879-1924. *Parliaments, Estates & Representation, 15,* 143-157.

U.S. Bureau of Labor and Statistics. (1996, June). A cps supplement for testing methods of collecting racial and ethnic information: May 1995 (BLS Statistical Notes Publication No. 40). Retrieved February 15, 2004 from: http://www.bls.census.gov/cps/racethn/1995/stat40rp.htm.

U.S. Census Bureau (1988, October). How census information is used. Census '90 press release. U.S. Department of the Commerce. Washington, DC.

U.S. Census Bureau (2002, April). *Measuring America: The decennial censuses from 1790 to 2000.* (Publication No. POL/02-MA). Retrieved January 26, 2004 from U.S. Census Bureau Reports Online: http://www.census.gov/prod/www/abs/genref.html.

U.S. Census Bureau (2000, May). *History and organization of the census* (Publication No. CFF-4). Retrieved January 26, 2004 from Factfinder for the Nation Online: http://landview.census.gov/population/www/cen2000/briefs.html.

U.S. Census Bureau (1997, July). Recommendations from the interagency committee for the review of the racial and ethnic standards to the office of management and budget concerning changes to standards for the classification of federal data on race and ethnicity (3110-01). Retrieved January 26, 2004, from U.S. Census Bureau online: http://www.census.gov/population/www/socdemo/race/Directive_15.html.

U.S. Census Bureau (1997, August). Report to congress. The plan for census 2000. Department of Commerce. Retrieved March 3, 2004, from U.S. Census Bureau online: http://www.census.gov/main/www/stat_activities.html.

U. S. Constitution, Art. I, § 2.

Yamashita, R. C. & Park, P. (1985). The politics of race: The open door, ozawa and the case of the japanese in america. *Review of Radical Political Economics, 17*(3), 135-156.

Zimmerman, M. A. (1990). Taking aim on empowerment research: On the distinction between psychological and individual conceptions. *American Journal of Community Psychology, 18,* 169-177.

Zimmerman, M. A. (1995). Psychology empowerment: Issues and illustrations. *American Journal of Community Psychology, 23,* 581-600.

Zinn, H. (2003). *A people's history of the united states: 1492-present.* New York: Harper Collins.

doi:10.1300/J137v15n04_08

Index

Page numbers followed by an *f* or *t* indicate figures or tables.

T - #0572 - 101024 - C0 - 212/152/9 - PB - 9780789036476 - Gloss Lamination